DANCING
IN THE
NARROWS

Cat,
Here's to
Hope and resilience —
Anna Penenberg

DANCING IN THE NARROWS

A Mother-Daughter Odyssey
Through Chronic Illness

ANNA PENENBERG

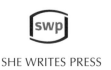

SHE WRITES PRESS

Published 2020
Printed in the United States of America
ISBN: 978-1-63152-838-5
ISBN: 978-1-63152-839-2
Library of Congress Control Number: 2020900785

For information, address:
She Writes Press
1569 Solano Ave #546
Berkeley, CA 94707

Interior design by Tabitha Lahr

She Writes Press is a division of SparkPoint Studio, LLC.

To my beloved daughters, Cayla and Dana,
who inspire me beyond words.

When Dana was twelve, I went with her sixth-grade class to Death Valley on a camping trip to study its unique geology. Fifty-mile-an-hour winds greeted us as we unpacked and set up tents. We ate with sand on our plates, slept with the moon, and rose with the sun. The desert spoke to us each day as we visited the fascinating geological features. On our last day, we explored the Eureka Dunes. When we arrived, the kids split up into groups, and I led one group on a trek into the monolithic sand formations, while Dana went off with a group led by another parent, seizing the chance to be on her own. Lagging behind my group on the way back, I glanced up toward the ridge of the dunes, and there, a silhouette against the sun, running like the wind across the spine of the world, arms flying, feet splayed like a dancer, was my daughter. I will see this image for the rest of my life.

AUTHOR'S NOTE

Many people today are affected by chronic illness, and Lyme disease is epidemic. I want to acknowledge all those, and their families, who have struggled to find a diagnosis, medical care, and/or alternatives that provide effective treatment options.

This memoir is a personal story and not intended to educate the reader about how to treat Lyme disease. I have used fictitious names and modified identifying details to protect the privacy of the doctors and practitioners with whom we worked.

CONTENTS

⊷⊷✖⊷⊷

PROLOGUE

Butty

What the caterpillar calls the end of the world,
the master calls a butterfly.

—Richard Bach

In 1997 Dana was seven years old and her sister, Cayla, nine. We were giggling and learning about life at our big house on Stone Canyon Road in Los Angeles, where the days were always sunny. Friends and their children came over to play. There were naked water fights on the lawn, hands covered in cornstarch "goop," and cherry tomatoes popping into mouths. Toy cars roamed our patio's adobe tiles, and easels held bright colors of paint, brushes, and large pads of paper. Our home was a haven for creativity, wildness, and discovery.

I planted a sunflower playhouse for my children in our vegetable garden. I had seen a picture of a garden "house" made of full-grown, six-foot-tall sunflower stalks with large yellow heads and spindly pole bean plants winding through them with big fat green beans dangling. I loved having a vegetable garden outside the kitchen, which made it easy for fresh picking and quick cooking. My two adventuresome girls played outside on both sides of our kitchen, which had plenty of windows for keeping an eye on them. Cayla moved swiftly and laughed loudly, while Dana had a slow grace and was quieter and more patient. They were inseparable.

Our sunflower house grew from the tiny seeds I painstakingly planted. As the stalks rose, I began weaving the pole beans through, except in the twelve-inch gap I left for the entry door. I entered it on my knees, slinking like a cat, smelling the musky green stalks, crawling all the way inside for secret meetings with my girls. It grew taller and taller, smiles bursting in yellow, seeded faces, giving hours of pleasure to two little girls hiding in living nature.

It was there that they became interested in caterpillars. They found them on the milkweed just outside the sunflower house. One day at the toy store we visited regularly, Dana found a cute little bughouse.

"I want this to put my bugs in!" she exclaimed.

"Me too!" said Cayla.

Holding her bughouse, Dana looked up at me and asked, "Mommy, can I have a pet caterpillar?"

"That's a wonderful idea! You know your book *The Very Hungry Caterpillar*? Remember that the caterpillar builds a cocoon and then it comes out as a butterfly?"

"I can't wait!" she shrieked, as she launched herself off the floor, landing in a joyous thud, over and over again.

Pretty soon we had two caterpillar pets living in clear plastic bughouses in our house. Every day the girls fed them with fresh water and leaves. Every day there was something new to see.

"Mommy, he ate the whole leaf I put in there!"

This entry into the world of a small being who naturally transforms itself from one who crawls to one who flies, suddenly became important to me. I knew that by witnessing this we would be changed forever. Nature was teaching us something. I thought of all the things I wanted my daughters to learn: to enjoy nature, to engage with living things, to understand the natural world is about relationships. I was grateful that nature, through the caterpillar to butterfly transformation, was exemplifying the process that occurs inside of us as we grow through life.

It was time to provide for the cocoon, so each girl selected a twig and placed it inside her box. We waited for the miracle. Finally, Dana's caterpillar formed a cocoon one night when we weren't watching. It looked like beige cotton candy, about an inch long and wrapped tightly around the twig at one end.

"Mommy, nothing's happening. How long will it take to be a butterfly?"

"Around two weeks," I read.

Before I could stop her, Dana reached into the bughouse, clasped her fingers around the twig, and lifted it out.

"Oh my! We don't want to disturb him while he's sleeping. He needs more time to grow into a beautiful butterfly. Let me help you put him back in his house until he's ready." My hand moved light as a feather as I took hold of the twig, cocoon hanging, and settled it back safely.

"I just want to see the butterfly!"

"I know, honey," I soothed.

Off she ran out the door into the garden just as the sprinklers went on. I could hear her shrill giggles.

Delicious summer days went by and soon it was time for our family vacation, a trip across the country to visit my in-laws and attend a family camp.

Dana protested, "Mommy, we can't leave our cocoons here. What if the butterflies hatch? We have to take them with us!"

Realizing that we were deep into the transformation of chrysalis to butterfly, and that they would die if we left them indoors for two weeks, I felt determined to take them. We packed and prepared and still both caterpillars were hanging in brown pouches from their twigs in the little bughouses. We smuggled both pets onto the plane heading cross-country from Los Angeles to New Jersey. I had no idea if Dana and Cayla's not-yet-butterflies would survive the altitude and change of air quality, but we continued with all the faith that magic can inspire in little girls' minds.

All went well, and we (including the butterfly cocoons) settled into Grandmother's spotlessly clean 1960s retirement community apartment. We placed the plastic butterfly houses on the kitchen counter in a protected place. On our first morning there, we went outside to gather fresh leaves from the abundant maple trees. All seemed undisturbed as we looked into the bughouses, anxious about how much longer it would take for the chrysalises to become butterflies. On the third day, we got a surprise.

During the night, one of the butterflies had broken out of its cocoon with the top of the plastic house still on, causing moisture to deform one of the wings and keep it from opening fully. Even though the top wing on her right side was folded, she was strikingly beautiful as a newborn. Her good wing was rich in amber tones and outlined in white-speckled black edges. We gathered around, peering into the small box with this magical creature inside.

Because "Butty" couldn't fly, we immediately became her family, knowing she could never leave home. The girls figured out how to get her to walk on plants so she could flick her long, thick tongue out and back to take in nourishment. What a treasure it was to watch the life of a butterfly up close!

"Mommy, look at her little tongue. I think she likes these flowers!"

It was a delicate operation holding the box steady as Butty tiptoed lightly out of the box onto a plant. She would walk up the stalk and into the flowers. The girls were mesmerized. Being able to watch her up close, knowing she couldn't take off, was a special honor. Butty liked a big blue hydrangea in the backyard, and we almost lost sight of her in the dewy petals. After feeding, she would tickle the leaves, her wings swaying as she walked back down the stalk and into her box house.

Our time in New Jersey was coming to a close. We were planning to drive to upstate New York for a week of family camp. Dana and Cayla cried out, "What are we going to do, Mommy? We can't leave Butty!" I fashioned a home for her out of a large shoebox comfortable enough for her to travel in, and off we went in our rental car.

From the back seat I heard Dana say, "Butty, look, here are my favorite books. Do you want me to read to you?"

Cayla whispered sweetly to her, "I'm glad you're with us even though I miss my cat, Fluffy."

Butty traveled well, landing in our dorm room closet for the week along with the other plastic bug home still housing the unhatched cocoon. The camp had a large and inviting vegetable garden, big enough for the girls to hide between the long rows, and perfect for Butty. The girls made many trips to this garden, taking their beloved butterfly out in the daylight and placing her gently on different plants. Butty was totally dependent on them, and they were fascinated. At night they put a light fabric over her little shoebox so she could sleep undisturbed.

During the fifth day there, Butty wasn't acting like her usual self. She seemed slower and less interested in flicking out her long tongue for nourishment, worrying the girls. So I explained that butterflies have short lives. I checked on her in the afternoon and discovered she was lifeless. She'd had a long life in butterfly years. We took Butty's wilted body outside and buried it with a prayer. Sweat rolled down my back from the humidity, and Dana's tears soaked my blouse. We had been suspended in time while a fascinating connection into the world of tiny beings and plants took over our hearts. Butty had left us with a deep love of the natural world.

A few years later when Dana was ten, she and I spent a summer on the Hampshire College campus in western Massachusetts. I was in a practitioner training program there, studying Body-Mind Centering, a somatic discipline I would later use in my healing practice with infants and children.

I attempted to make the youth program on campus sound appealing to Dana by telling her she would be going to "day camp" while I was in class. She shot back with, "Mom, I'm old enough to be on my own. I don't want to go to day camp!"

"What will you do when I'm in class?"

"I'll go scootering . . . and sometimes I'll sit at the back of your class and knit my scarf."

"Hmm . . . Okay, but you have to check in with me so I know where you are. Keep track of the time on your watch."

"Yay!" She did a little happy dance.

Dana spent her time among the trees, gardens, and grass areas of the vast campus. There she found herself again in the lap of nature. She spent her time admiring each leaf in the vegetable gardens and each petal on the flowers surrounding the buildings.

We had lunch together every day, and one day after we'd devoured our ice cream cones, Dana grabbed my hand and exclaimed with glee, "Come with me! I want to show you my garden. I know every plant in there, and I'm watching them grow and blossom!"

I can still hear her laughter ringing through the New England foliage as she rode her scooter over the dirt paths on campus. She was free.

It may have been in the vegetable garden that a tiny tick crawled onto her leg, embedded its teeth in her tender skin, and drew her blood into its mouth. I never imagined that a tiny insect could, some years later, make her life unbearable with discomfort. Nature isn't all benevolent. There are deaths and killings and pathogenic takeovers. There are species vying for survival and borrowing bodies to carry them around. So it is with the Ixod tick that can breed Lyme spirochetes in its belly and then suck the blood of a young girl to nourish itself, leaving behind spirochetes to thrive and multiply in their new host.

PART ONE

CHAPTER ONE

Movement in My Life

*If you don't have self-reliance, what do you have? You can
cross the mountains, the oceans, the tragedies, the difficulties,
the responsibilities, with only one thing, self-reliance. Fear not,
my dear ones; the antidote for fear is self-reliance.*

— Yogi Bhajan

As a girl I reveled in moving, dancing, twirling; I never
wanted to be constricted, held back, or forced to be still.
My mother accommodated my passion by installing a ballet bar
along the entire length of the long corridor off the bedrooms
in our Spanish-style Los Angeles home.

Pirouetting into the hallway from my bedroom, dressed
in a black leotard and pink tights, I announced, "I'm shutting
the doors to the hall!" My corridor of freedom. Just then, Jain,
my younger sister, darted out of her bedroom. Imperiously, I
turned on her: "Jain, it's my turn on the ballet bar!"

She pouted and whined, "I want to dance too."

I paused for effect, considered her for a moment, and then gave my orders: "Follow me! We're doing leaps up and down the hallway." Off we leapt past three generations of family photos.

Tovya, my older sister, peered down the hallway from the living room. I leapt in her direction. She was louder and more talkative, and generally called the shots, but this was *my* corridor of freedom. "Hey!" I said, knowing she might take over. "I'm leading, you can follow. Now we are going to do a grand plié on the ballet bar. I'll be in front, Jain in the middle, and you at the end."

•••••••••••∴•••••••••••

When I was seventeen, I entered San Diego State College to study dance and psychology. I was living in the brand-new freshman dorm, a nine-story tower called "El Conquistador." It was so new that they had just paved the parking area and hadn't finished installing the parking lot lights.

On September 26, 1970, the "Laguna Fire" flared up and burned for eight days, turning the sky black. It ended up scorching 175,425 acres.

"Let's go up to the ninth floor and look at the fire!" someone shouted.

Even though we had watched the fire from there before, my roommate, Rhonda, and I flew up the stairs. She said, "I've seen people who don't live here up on the ninth floor looking at the fire."

I nodded. "Yeah. . . . It's so weird not being able to see the sky." I had just left home for the first time in my life, and the apocalyptic experience of being engulfed by smoke felt scary. I didn't have my bearings yet. Everything was new for me.

We reached the balcony and hung back from the small crowd. I looked around and saw our small group of new friends from the dorm. We walked over to join them, and as I got closer, I noticed a tall guy I didn't know. He was a bit older than us, with blond hair, a short beard, and a cast up to the elbow of one arm.

"Hi, my name is Karl. I just came up to see the fire. What a great vantage point!" He seemed nice.

I asked, "Do you go to San Diego State?"

"No, I live in the area. I'm out of school."

"What happened to your arm?"

"I broke it falling off my bicycle, but the cast should come off soon."

Looking out at the sky, I shouted, "Rhonda, check out the sunset! It looks like a red ball against the dark sky. Really eerie!"

Eventually, our group, with Karl tagging along, trooped downstairs to the common room. A girl named Sally asked, "Does anyone have any food? Munchies?"

Mark answered, "No. Let's go to the store and get chips, dip, and some cookies!"

That was when Karl spoke up. "I have a car—I'll drive." We pooled our money together, but I was the only one who volunteered to make the trip with Karl. He seemed friendly enough, and my new gang of friends seemed to accept him, so I didn't feel weird going with him. I was dating a boy I knew from temple in LA, and did not view Karl as anything other than one of the group.

We walked out of the dorm toward the dark parking lot. Karl opened the door to his van and let me in on the passenger side. Then he got in to drive, but before he started the car, he leaned over and tried to kiss me. I recoiled and flattened myself against the door, but he kept at it. *This is so embarrassing! I'm not even interested in him.*

I kept protesting and dodging his lips. He got angry, grabbed me roughly by the arms, hoisted me over the seat, and threw me into the back of the van. He crawled in back and began beating me with his cast. He whaled on me, landing bone-bruising blows. My feet hit hard between his legs. I fought to save my life. The more I fought, the more aggressive he became.

"HELP! HEEEEELP! HEEEEEELP!" My voice sounded like ripped paper. He pounded harder. I lost consciousness, and he took me aggressively, tearing my sweet pink summer dress. I woke up, and while he was in the front seat doing something I couldn't see, I groped around frantically until I found the sliding-door handle. I managed somehow to slide it open, and I bolted, running as fast as my shocked and brutalized body could go.

I reached the front door of the dorm and pounded furiously. Somebody finally opened it, and I pushed my way inside. Turning around, I caught a glimpse of Karl's face. He had caught up with me. Capturing his eyes in mine, I rasped, "I didn't know people like you existed!" The heavy metal door slammed in his face.

• • • • • • • •᠁• • • • • • • •

The summer following my first year of college, I landed back in LA. I was living with my parents and working as a waitress at Marie Callender's Restaurant & Bakery. Mom and Dad were thrilled to have leftover pie fillings for breakfast.

On my off hours I hung out with my old friend Deb, one of the very few I had told about the rape. She was worried about me and invited me to go with her to a psychodrama session. The sessions were led by a charismatic, thirtysomething psychotherapist named Michael, and these weekly group meetings were held in his living room. One person volunteered to work out his or her issues each week. At each session, all the people present were called on to act out roles from the volunteer's life. One evening I was asked to play the role of someone's angry mother, which powerfully affected us all. After a few weeks of going regularly, Deb asked, "Can I tell Michael about your rape?"

Reluctantly, I said, "I guess so." I'd kept the rape a secret from almost everyone.

At the next session, all of us were huddled on the rose carpet in Michael's living room. I sat like a coiled snake.

Michael asked, "Anna, would you like to work tonight?"

All jittery inside, with cold hands and a pale face, I croaked, "Okay."

Michael placed his arm lightly on my back to stabilize me, and asked, "May I tell the group about your difficult experience almost a year ago?"

"Yes." I was terrified to reveal what had happened, but it was so horrible to keep it stuffed down inside of me. The few others I'd told so far hadn't thought I needed help, not the nurse at student health services, not even my mom.

"Anna had a violent and invasive experience. She was raped about a year ago." It almost felt good to hear him say that, to hear the truth spoken out loud.

Michael directed the group: "Form a circle around Anna." Shuffling bodies formed a large circle around me. I was the deer in headlights.

He told them, "Move tightly together," and asked me, "Is there anything you want to share, Anna?"

"Yes. . . . He had a cast on his arm and he beat me."

Sighs, exhales, watery eyes in the room. *They know it was bad.*

Michael faced me with his hands on my shoulders. "Your job is to break out of the circle." He looked at the others and said, "Your job is to prevent her from getting out."

The room shrunk to the size of a small tiger, and I began to panic with full-blown shivers reverberating through my body.

"Anna, you have to find a way to get out. You are not held hostage anymore—you can do something different."

I could feel the cold van, the dark, the beating of my heart, racing to save my life. I was almost paralyzed. My reality blended memory and the present moment. My hands became claws. I was enraged, pulsing, hot, a human knife. I reached between two people and pulled, trying to pry their hands apart, but nothing budged. I scanned the circle for another weak opening. People's eyes locked on me to engage my courage. I dove under. Bodies stopped me. I ran and leapt high. The circle buckled but managed to ensnare me and toss me back into the center. I went to the side of the ring, as if I were in a wrestling match. I hated each and every person in the circle. I ripped them apart with my eyes. My pounding heart was making enough blood pulse for someone twice my size. Sweat poured down my face. I waited for surprise to raise my chances, then cut into a crevasse in the wall, my body the knife. I made it to the other side—a sutured wound.

CHAPTER TWO

Becoming Myself

Obstacles don't have to stop you. If you run into a wall,
don't turn around and give up. Figure out how to climb it,
go through it, or work around it.

— Michael Jordan

I transferred to UC Berkeley in my junior year and spent one, less than happy quarter there before I applied for a transfer to UCLA to become part of their renowned Dance Department. However, I was denied admission, so I set up a meeting with the head of the department, Alma Hawkins.

I sat stiffly across from the formidable grande dame, who was renowned for her understanding of movement as an art form as well as a statement of self. I was primly dressed in a gray floral silk dress that had been my great grandmother's because I wanted to look professional. I gazed into Alma's clear and perceptive eyes and spoke with conviction: "I think you've made a mistake. I have too many units to transfer, but I *know* I belong here."

A sparrow landed on the windowsill. I went on, "I need to be in *this* dance department. Its philosophy of nonverbal expression is what I believe in. I want to discover myself in this art form." I watched for her reaction. She took me seriously and asked a few questions about my previous experience.

"I did not fit into the dance department at Berkeley. It was too focused on Martha Graham technique and performance. I could not discover my own movement. UCLA is where I need to do my work." I wasn't able to decipher how she was responding to me. The sparrow took off. My nerves wanted to kick in, but I held them back. All I had left to say was one thing.

"You must make this happen!" I used up all my confidence in that one sentence. I cannot remember anything that was said after that, but Alma made it happen.

<hr/>

I loved my experience at UCLA. Our dance department occupied an entire two-story building that was once the women's gym. It came complete with lockers, showers, and a redwood sauna. I did my best thinking while sweating in the dark after dance class. All dance majors were exposed to the style and philosophy of visiting dance companies, including José Limón, Merce Cunningham, Pilobolus, Martha Graham, Alvin Ailey, and others. We trained with them in master classes and watched their performances at Royce Hall. I couldn't have been happier.

One day in technique class, I had an epiphany. It was 1:00 p.m. Tuesday in the UCLA Dance Department studio A, Sharon's class. I liked her. She was sharp, concise in her movement, agile, and elflike, and could make up and memorize long phrases of movements. Because she thrived on small detailed gestures and quick locomotion footwork, I found her choreography difficult. This particular Tuesday I was grieving the end of a relationship and overwhelmed with homework. I'd put all that aside and showed up for class. We warmed up as usual.

"Remember the exercises we've been doing? Start with the floor stretches." I sat down at floor level with both legs straight out in front and began to bow forward. As my chest went up and down, I felt grateful to be stretching. It was years before yoga would become a common practice for me, but I knew stretching, breathing, and focusing on the exercises would bring me back from the mad details of my student life.

Sharon stood before us. "Class, I will demonstrate today's movement phrase. Then we'll connect it to the other phrases we've learned, and you will know the first section of my new choreography!"

She began modeling the new phrase. *Oh my God, another tricky mind-bending series of movements that are built for her body and not mine.* It was like speaking in a foreign language. I relentlessly complied, perfecting my movements, waving my arms, making light, quick shuffles with my feet, executing a wide turn and a leap that sent me across the room.

"Okay, everyone, let's go one at a time." We were lining up at one corner, ready to dart across the studio diagonally, but suddenly I wanted to sit down. My stomach roiled with grief. All of me wanted stillness. I watched the girl before me prance her way across the room in what looked like a joyous state. *My turn.* I heard the live piano start and launched myself at the perfect beat, setting out across the floor. All eyes were on me. As I danced, my internal feelings mushroomed. The grief escalated and the urge to stop became paralyzing. I was halfway across the floor. *Can't everyone see I'm faking it? It isn't me, this movement. I'm pretending.* I felt transparent. I pushed through and let my body continue to perform the phrase against my own mood.

What movement does my body want *to do? What would it look like if I moved my grief?* I became powerfully aware of movement as expression, and aware that movement moves feeling. *I can make it to the far corner. I'm almost there!* When I reached the wall, I leaned all my weight against it, trying not to cry. Inside I was spinning with the challenge of fathoming my new awareness. The music stopped. All eyes turned to the next dancer, and I was revolutionized. I would never override my feelings willingly again. I did not like it. I felt separate from myself. I had, in that moment, realized my desire to become a practitioner who used body movement for healing and self-expression.

<hr/>

I moved to Sonoma County in Northern California when I graduated from UCLA. Being in Sonoma, a rural wine region with rolling hills and a lush landscape, gave me the chance to experience country living. The idea of really being on my own frightened me as much as it excited me. I rented a room not far from my younger sister, Jain, who was attending college there.

The Sonoma Mountain Outdoor Experience program was looking for youth counselors in my age range. Mondays, Wednesdays, and Fridays, I took curious eight- and nine-year-olds on a four-hour hike around the Sonoma County Preserve. We would collect specimen bugs, touch moss, and spot small scurrying animals and overhead birds.

"Look here, everyone." The kids gathered around me. "What do you see on this wire fence?" A large hawk had died with his wingspan fully open. The kids were amazed, horrified, and fascinated.

"Is he dead?" Mari asked.

"Yes. This is a red-tailed hawk. How do you think he died?"

"He hit the fence," a tall boy named Eli shouted.

"That's possible. It looks like he may have had a problem and didn't see the wire. In nature, animals die and become food for others. Soon he will provide for the crows. He may have been old—these hawks can live up to twelve years. That's older than you are!"

"He won't be buried?"

"No, Douglas," I replied gently, as I knew his grandfather had just died. "Out here, nature takes its course."

By day I was content with my life and my work with the children, but when I was alone at night, the anxiety of adulthood, of all the choices I knew I'd have to make, overwhelmed me. I found myself eating whole pies in the privacy of my room. I loved crust, and the more I ate, the more comforted I felt. I also felt bloated, numb, and slowed down, which muted the anxiety.

I overate wheat in whatever blissful form it came in. For dinner I would consume sandwiches, pot pies, or pizza, and then pie for dessert. Sometimes I even craved Wonder Bread! While stuffing it in my grateful, salivating mouth, I wondered about my future, my identity, my ability to be self-sustaining. Maybe I was scared to be alone; maybe I was scared a man would hurt me again. I knew I was still healing.

I resisted my compulsion by refusing to keep pie in the house. That meant that often, late at night, I'd have to drive to the closest convenience store and buy the most natural, unnatural frozen apple pie I could find. At my apartment I'd heat it in the oven, drenching the room in the delectable aroma of sweet apple and yeasty crust. I'd sit in my old, stained loveseat with the bubbling pie perched on my chipped coffee table and dig in.

Sticky, previously frozen apples dripped off my fork as I aimed for my mouth. Bite after bite. I always attempted to eat only one pie slice, but I never cut the pie into pieces, so in the end the whole pie was mine. After my gluttony I knew sleep would come with a heavy stomach, and the buzzing panic would give way to murky dreams that would be gone by morning.

⁕⁕⁕⁕⁕⁕⁕⁕⁖⁕⁕⁕⁕⁕⁕⁕

That summer I took an intensive dance therapy course in the Blanche Evan Method. Blanche sashayed into the dance studio wearing purple pants, an orange blouse, a twisted silk purple scarf at her neck, and silver jewelry on her ears and wrists. She was a dancer who had studied Adlerian "individual psychology." Fascinated, I was excited to learn how to dance into the psychological.

"Find your place in the room." We were in the gym at Sonoma State College, a vast and unstructured room with a hardwood floor. I located myself next to the heavy velvet curtain and sat down cross-legged. "Imagine a memory that felt good to you. Go through the motions of whatever you need to enact this, to discover what lies underneath."

I sat imagining. Finally, I felt the urge to create. I saw a kitchen in my mind and built it through movement: the stove, the counter, the refrigerator, the sink and cupboards. It was a country kitchen made of pine cupboards, painted white floorboards, and golden handmade ceramic dishes. I took out a large, white mixing bowl and began to make cookie batter. I knew it by heart.

First I measured the three-fourths cup of granulated sugar, then packed the three-fourths cup of brown sugar, mashed a cup of butter, added a teaspoon of vanilla and an egg, and stirred vigorously. Then I added the two and one-fourth cups of flour, the teaspoon of baking soda, salt, nuts, and a whole package of semisweet chocolate chips. Creating a lumpy, sweet, thick mound of delight, I scooped spoonfuls onto the cookie sheet. I heated the oven to 350 degrees and waited for it to be hot.

Blanche came by to check in on me. Her short gray hair and glasses framed a penetrating view of my experience. "What are you doing and how is it going?"

"I'm baking chocolate chip cookies. I've gotten as far as making the batter and scooping the dollops onto the cookie sheet. I'm in a place of nourishment, no worries—like with my grandma Betty in her kitchen, baking."

"Keep it going."

I baked more cookies than I could count over the next two hours. I couldn't stop. It was a private heaven for my psyche. Nothing else in the world was going on. Blanche came to me several more times.

"Find your motivation." I kept going into my private kitchen and creating the food I needed most to enliven my life. My sweetness, my grandmother love, my own expanding hope—all went into the uncooked batter. The cookies would come out freshly born, crunchy and tender inside, chocolate bits slightly melting in my mouth. The perfection of pleasure.

CHAPTER THREE

I Am the Mover

The good life is one inspired by love and
guided by knowledge.

— Bertrand Russell

That fall I entered one of UCLA's first graduate classes in dance therapy, headed by Irma Dosamantes-Beaudry, PhD, a dance therapist and psychoanalyst. We were a small group of eight students and became very close. During my last year of the program, the VA hospital's drug addiction rehab program offered an internship for one student in our class. Irma chose me.

Off we went together for the first session, where I had to lead the men in front of my professor. After that I was on my own, hoping my training and the private supervision I was lucky to have with Irma each week was enough.

Arriving for the second session, I entered the large, square industrial room that housed the drug rehab program. The men were congregated at the back. They had already stacked the chairs to the side and taken their shoes off. They knew from the first session that we would be sitting in a circle on the floor. I looked around at the warm wood floor and steel-barred windows and gestured for the men to join me on the floor. We sat in a circle, and I said, "Use your arms to make a movement that shows how you're feeling today."

A young, tall, thin black man towered over the group from his perch on the top of the tallest column of stacked chairs. He said, "I'm James and I feel fine, little Miss Bo Peep!" My blond hair flowed over my slim shoulders, which were clothed in a plain white button-down blouse. I grasped the irony of my situation. I was a white, middle-class college girl attempting to help these young men, Vietnam vets who had seen and done things I didn't know anything about.

"Thank you, James. I see you appreciate a high vantage point. We are here when you want to come down and join us."

Next, Doug sheepishly swung his arms around and politely welcomed the "lady." I was to be protected. Tension was high in the room, like a large, stretched-to-the-max rubber band. I honestly couldn't see how I could help these men, but I firmly believed in using movement for expression. I never would have guessed that my first clients would be streetwise men who had been to war.

••••••••••••••••••••

I proceeded. Our group bonded. I reminded them of sister, mother, and grandmother, despite my young age. They began to feel safe opening up and sharing their stories. We would close our sessions with hands held clear around the circle. There were always soft eyes and a few tears.

James held his place on top of the chairs for a couple of weeks, but eventually came down to join us. I took on a few individual cases during that time, and the VA program wanted me to see James. I had never spent time with someone who had only experienced living through drugs. He said, "As soon as I could walk, I would go to the fridge and fetch my mom's heroin for her." He had come a long way but had much to learn. I became his guide into the sober world.

We had been working together for about five months when, in one of our last sessions, he seemed troubled. As part of the rehab program, he had been spending several days a week at a job outside the VA hospital. James began to pace and pace and pace. I sat on the floor across from the windows. He wound around and around the room, stopping to look out the window into the city. With every round, more questions.

"What's it like to live every day without drugs? What do you do?"

I stumbled inside, knowing he needed modeling for a world he had never been in. "You get up and feed yourself a good breakfast, go to work, make good sober friends, and enjoy activities that do not involve drugs, like walking, reading, and seeing movies. You will have to let go of your old habits. Friends will not be for drug connections."

He paced for the hour, asking and taking in. "What's it like to go to the movies? I mean, what would the whole evening be like?"

"You could go with a friend to a little restaurant for pizza and talk, then walk to the movie theater, buy tickets, and go in."

"I've never sat around and talked with anyone. At least, not if it wasn't a therapy group in the program. I wouldn't know what to say."

"Let's practice."

I worried about leaving the program, and hoped it would come at a time when James could sustain his new sober life. I was his only close-up example of an adult living without drugs. I cared about the young man he could be, with the dear, sweet soul inside. I wanted him to live his life out of danger and addiction. I was his family.

• • • • • • • • • • • • • • • • • •

After graduate school, at the age of twenty-four, I was hired as the Alhambra Psychiatric Hospital's dance therapist. I worked there for three years, during which time I obtained a California State psychotherapy license. I was originally slated to run a group for adolescent girls, but in the end and against my wishes, I became the facilitator of the adolescent boys' group as well. I didn't have brothers, so I was concerned I would be out of my element with the boys. In both the boys' and girls' groups, I was going to be dealing with teen bullies and kids with street sense, drug habits, ADHD, schizophrenia, and anxiety.

I dressed in loose pants, low-heeled shoes, and a dark jacket, my straight blond hair clipped together in a low ponytail. I was careful to project a nonthreatening, if not somewhat androgynous image.

Into the fire I went:

"Hey, Tom, my girlfriend here is fuckin' awesome!" Referring to me.

"Yeah, Jim, I just farted. I think she can tell."

"Tom . . . jeez. Let's get Greg over here to torment him."

"Wha' the fuck, Jim, you slimy creature!"

There was a locker room smell of sweaty socks. Hormones raged. I intervened. "Okay, let's gather into a circle and sit down." The rest of the hour became a contest to see how many swear words and gross images they could insert between the tasks of the session. I felt like a skinny competitor in a sumo wrestling ring.

I came prepared to the second session with a large, white exercise ball and plenty of chalk. "Gather up, guys. Tom and Jim in the back, that means you too. Yep, the front of the room, facing the blackboard. Okay, who wants to do the writing?"

They were calm, waiting to see what I was going to do.

"Thank you, Scott, for volunteering. You are going to take this chalk and write down the words we tell you."

I turned to face the boys. "The next ten minutes are for all the words you can think of that I wouldn't want to hear, and words you are not supposed to use on the ward."

Silence.

"And . . . go! The clock is ticking."

They sprang into action, and even the most reserved in the bunch yelled words for the slam board: "Asshole!" "Fuck you!" "Bastard!" "Son of a Bitch!" "Cunt!"

This became our ritual every session. Ten free minutes for slam words, loud laughter, grossness, and anxiousness. I loved this time when all hell could carefully break loose, and I would become part of the group.

I also instituted something I called the big ball exercise. I had the boys line up in front of the side wall, and said, "You may punch or throw the ball at the wall. Your task is to say one word or sentence that you need to express, and then put your feelings into the ball. This can be someone's name, something you never got to say, how you're feeling today."

"Anything?" asked Jim.

"Yes, but this is without swear words, and you will need to be a little thoughtful. The person using the ball will be heard and get everyone's support."

Scott was at the head of the line. "This is for my mean dad." He used his open hand to punch the ball, and it cracked into the sidewall and bounced off in powerful flight across the room. I shuddered, wondering if the mirror would come down and I would lose my job.

"Neeext! Keep your place in line," I instructed. Everyone who wanted a turn had one.

Little Bob was hesitant and refused. I reassured him. "You can move the ball any way you want, even tap it lightly, or you can take a turn in our next meeting."

Words came toward Little Bob from all sides of the room. "Go for it, Bob!" "We got your back!" "Do it for yourself!" Little Bob sauntered forward, holding the ball across his small body, and said, "I miss my mom," and grievingly gave it a push toward the wall.

Larry grabbed the ball on the rebound and put his arm around Little Bob. "Bob, don't worry, you'll get over it even though it is hard." Larry's mother had also left him at an early age. I had a soft spot for Little Bob, so raw from his loss. *How could a mother leave her child? How could she let him feel unwanted?*

* * * * *

Wendy came to Alhambra Psychiatric Hospital not long after birthing her third child. She arrived for her first meeting nicely dressed in khaki pants topped with a floral cotton blouse, suffering from postpartum depression.

I took Wendy to a treatment room in the adult wing of the hospital. Breathing shallowly, she had a whisper-soft voice. "I have three children. My husband is taking care of them, my parents too." I watched her and couldn't find any emotion in her body or words—no longing, no missing her little ones, her husband, her life. She continued in a monotone, "I need to get well to help my husband. He is so nice." I wondered if she had this sentence on automatic programming.

I was fairly naïve about the biochemistry involved in the hormonal storm of postpartum depression, but cared about her recovery. As I worked with her, I became aware that she had suicidal thoughts. I wanted to see her return home and mother her children. Her newborn baby wasn't bonding with an absent mother. We bonded, however, quietly and without much feeling, but at least she felt safe with me.

One cold winter day Wendy and I had an hour together in a much smaller room, which was long and narrow. It was more private, with a modest window facing the back lawn. There were no chairs, so she slumped to the floor.

"I don't feel like moving."

"I see." I couldn't let her sit around and mumble any longer; I almost went into the fog with her. I wanted to scream, shake her loose, find where the dying ended. We sat in silence while I combed my creativity into a brave intervention.

"Okay. You rest for ten minutes." She seemed perplexed as everyone else wanted her to snap out of her endless fatigue and despondency. "I'll just sit here with you in silence." Over in the far corner, I saw the props stashed for occupational therapy. A jump rope, red and green fabric, pillows—these stood out for me. I needed to find a way to engage her. After the ten minutes I said, "I'll be getting up now."

No answer.

I set out the fabric as a line across the middle of the narrow room and gathered the pillows and rope. Holding on to the jump rope, I offered her one handle end. "Hold on for your life!" She barely wrapped her hand around it. In a kind voice I said, "Do you want to live? Do you?"

"I want to see my husband and my children again."

"Do you want to live?"

"I don't know."

"Hold on, because this is your life and it might fall out of your hands!" I increased the tension on the rope with minimal strength. She almost lost the handle.

"Hold on, because this represents your life, and you might have to fight for it."

She just barely hung on. I'd seen this in children; when they are screaming protests, part of them wants to stop. I stood up and explained the formation I had made on the floor. "The red and green line separates the area of death from the area of life. You now sit on the side of death. If you desire your life, you will have to find a way over the line."

"I don't want to."

"Your children, Alice, Max, and Olivia, are on the side of life. Benjamin, your husband, is on the side of life, your parents, your friends. The side of death is empty, dark, lonely."

Silence.

I placed a pile of pillows on the side of life and raised the challenge: "Do you want your children to be without a mother?" I stood, remaining on the side of life and pulling my end of the rope with some force, and saw her hand wrap itself around the handle. As I continued to pull, her other hand joined in. I paused, holding the rope tension. *Wow! She's responding. More of her is starting to fight.*

"How are you feeling over there in death?"

"I don't know."

"Yes, you do."

"I don't want to die."

"Okay. You are going to have to find a way over the line." I pulled harder. She leaned back and increased her grip on the handle.

"Hold on!" The harder I pulled, the more she engaged. Her feet dug into the rug, and she was up in a squat leaning against the wall. *I am like steel, and I won't stop until she gains her will to live!*

"I know you feel like giving up, it's been hard to be here. Don't think of anything but who you love!" More pull, more resistance. Wendy was still on the side of death. I saw her will strengthening.

"I am not letting go! I am holding you to engage in your life again!"

She winced, and tears formed while the darkness still held her.

"Make your choice! Choose what you really want!" My hands were hot and red, my eyes watered, but I pulled even harder. She stood in a wide stance and her eyes glared with a new, daring look. Could I hold on long enough for her to choose? She had become so good at giving up until I challenged her. I saw Wendy gather her strength, muscles activated from her toes to her shoulders, biceps appearing on her arms.

"What are you going to do?" I held the tension high and looked into her eyes.

Her face softened. She focused on the side of life and seemed to imagine moving. Wendy took a step forward and the rope pulled her over the line. The tension broke as she fell into the pillows on the side of life. I dropped down and held her. In a whisper I said, "You chose to live."

CHAPTER FOUR

Soul Retrieval

We must let go of the life we have planned,
so as to accept the one that is waiting for us.

—Joseph Campbell

Fifteen years later I was pregnant with my first daughter, Cayla. In my fourth month my sensitivity to odors became acute. While shopping at Whole Foods one day, I thought I might puke right there in the middle of the spice aisle after catching a whiff of the spices, even though they were all tightly sealed in their glass jars. A very pregnant woman passed me with her cart and noticed my distress. Through my nausea I uttered, "You look as if you are about to have a baby yourself."

She answered with excitement, "I'm due in two months."

I asked, "Did you have morning sickness?"

"Yes," she said, looking pained on my behalf. "It'll go away."

"I'm too nauseous to go to my Jane Fonda exercise classes for pregnant moms . . . and . . . feel really isolated."

She smiled kindly and offered, "Would you like to join me for a class at a yoga studio near here? It's led by a teacher named Gurmukh. We do gentle yoga exercises."

Grateful, I replied, "That sounds wonderful."

Four years later, while Cayla was in prekindergarten and my second daughter, two-year-old Dana, was off at preschool, I ventured out to take a Kundalini Yoga class with Guru Singh, a new teacher I'd recently found.

"Inhale, pull the locks . . . anus, sex organs, navel . . . hold! Exhale and reeelease."

Slowly drifting off into unconsciousness, I pulled myself back. I hated falling asleep between postures, but I'd done just that many times before.

After class I lay on my mat, dozing in a semiconscious state for a while, soaking up the comfort of Shavasana, also known as "corpse pose." I felt a tap on my shoulder. Guru Singh whispered, "Hello. I've watched you in class and see that you often fall asleep."

Embarrassed, I explained, "Yes, my little ones keep me awake at night."

"Would you like some help with that?"

A few days later I entered his private healing sanctuary, a cabin at the back of the property where he lived. It was a cave-like space hidden away from the left-brain world. Symbols, masks, and stones were deliberately strewn about the cabin. Messages filled the walls. Little shelves were lined with feathers, dried flowers, bones, and animal tokens. Native American articles, a dream catcher, and a large feather were placed with care. Ceremony took place here.

Guru Singh took my elbow and guided me to lie down face up on a cushiony, makeshift massage table. He put on a tape of Gurmukhi mantra chanting. He then placed two heavy onyx balls in my hands and wrapped me tightly in a bundle blanket. He began drumming, and I felt my body and mind soften as I relaxed deeply. My fingers softened around the cold stones, and my spine sunk down into the pillows. He covered my eyes with a soft cloth. All went dark.

Tensions in my body dissolved, and I retired inside to a nonthinking place, surrendering my conscious mind while the drumming took over. "Sound healing," he called it. I heard overtones and undertones and felt vibrations from a speaker under my body. I was dreaming, but awake. *A house of wisdom . . . a place to leave my stories behind, those which are in the way of my true identity.*

Time passed, easily thirty minutes. The drumming got louder and a short, sharp series of pounding rhythms brought me back to the room. I wiggled my hands and feet, awakening my "body glove," as Guru Singh liked to call it.

"I saw things vividly, like I was there and they were real."

"Good. They are real but not tangible."

"I thought I was going to learn how to stay awake in yoga class!"

"And I thought I would teach you how to be awake."

I had no difficulty "journeying," going into an altered state of consciousness, bringing in awareness beyond physical perception, and the drumming rhythms assisted in the process. I already meditated and thought in visual images, so this was familiar.

Guru Singh acknowledged, "You know this place." He opened me up to the magnitude of forces in the nonphysical by giving me a map: "The lower world is the animal instinctual realm, the middle world is a mirror of present time, the upper world has our guides and medicine healers."

While he trained me, I healed slowly, and during one of our early soul retrieval sessions, I received a bear as my power animal. A bear symbolizes strength, confidence, taking a stand against adversity, and the emergence of healing ability. Guru Singh "journeyed" to retrieve a soul part of mine, and after inviting my lost soul parts to return, he came upon an eighteen-month-old toddler hovering in a corner of a bathroom.

"I'm here to help you," Guru Singh said, offering her a glowing red ball of light. The child took the ball of light and held it to her chest. She said, "My mother is bleeding," then crawled into his arms and fell asleep. A seventeen-year-old part then appeared. Her blond hair was a mess and her body was shivering. She said, "I've been hurt." Guru Singh showed her the little one in his lap and invited her to sit with them. He placed his right hand on the back of her heart and let it heal. When they were ready to come "home," he blew them into my crown and solar plexus.

I awakened, my body vibrating from the sound current. Tears were spilling from my eyes as I said softly, "Thank you, Guru Singh. These are important pieces for me. My mother told me that she'd miscarried when I was a toddler, and when I was seventeen, I was raped."

I immediately felt lighter that day, my senses heightened. On my way home I noticed the sky had for the first time turned a real blue, and the trees lining the streets were a luminescent green. My heart sang inside!

Once a week for two years, I made the pilgrimage to Guru Singh's cabin, where he imparted the skills required to practice soul retrieval. Over time, healing took place in invisible ways. Beliefs changed, I saw things differently, and I was different with my new and freer confidence.

After I told my friend Hank about my soul retrieval training, he mentioned that his wife, Miranda, was suffering from terrible fatigue and was looking for help. I promptly recommended Sandra Ingerman's book *Soul Retrieval*. Miranda was the head of a busy family psychotherapy clinic but had taken a year off to deal with her health issues. She downed the book in two days and had Hank call me to ask where she could find a practitioner. I told him that I'd ask my teacher.

I explained to Guru Singh that my friend's wife had read Sandra's book and wanted to experience soul retrieval. I asked him if he would work with her.

He said, "You can see her."

I was a little taken aback and quickly responded, "I don't think I'm ready."

He said, "Yes, you are. You were here to learn. Now you're a healer."

My training was over, and I had my first client, a bright, knowledgeable, self-aware psychologist. With my ceremonial shawl (Jewish tallit), rattle, drumming tapes, cassette deck, and headphones, I set out not totally convinced I could do this soul retrieval healing. What if I blanked out? What if nothing came to me or I couldn't see anything in the imaginal realm?

Miranda greeted me at the front door of her gracious two-story Tudor-style home. She had short dark hair and an air of competence. A few years earlier I had attended a psychotherapy seminar she was hosting; now I was her healer. She led me into the den, and I grabbed a cushion off the couch for myself and laid out my shawl, a placeholder for spirit to find me.

I instructed Miranda to lie down and make herself comfortable. I took another cushion off the couch for her and said, "I'm going to wrap you in a blanket and place a cover over your eyes. Everything you know from being a therapist will not be relevant here."

"What do you mean?"

"We will not need information about your past and will not analyze what's going on with you. We're listening to guidance and calling back the places inside your being that have been lost during discomfort or danger. I'll journey quietly, retrieve your soul parts, and blow them into your solar plexus and the top of your crown."

"Okay. I read about that in Sandra's book."

"You can rest now and I'll call you back when I've returned your soul part." I lay down beside her, wrapped myself in a blanket, switched the drumming tape on, and went journeying for Miranda's soul parts. I secretly prayed that something would happen. I had lit a candle and set the intention for healing. *What if I don't see anything?*

A deer moved quickly through a stand of willow trees. Miranda's power animal, bringing the wisdom of grace moving through challenges. Soon I was in a field. A girl who told me she was eleven going on twelve ran by. I caught up with her. She was beside herself. "I'm unhappy. I don't feel good here."

"What do you need in order to come 'home'?"

"I want my family with me."

In this imaginary place, I called in her parents. They came willingly. She stopped running and joined her family, who were sitting around a picnic blanket laid out in the field.

"Are you ready to come 'home' now?"

"It's my birthday. I want to celebrate it at my own home."

The scene changed and I saw her enter a home somewhere in the Midwest. The table in the dining room was set with dessert dishes and a cake with twelve candles in the center. She walked into the room, which was now filled with her friends and family. She was beaming. I gave her a present wrapped in clear light. Twelve-year-old Miranda nodded yes. She was ready.

I leaned over forty-nine-year-old Miranda, lying quietly in her Los Angeles den, inhaled the soul part, and blew it into her crown and solar plexus. I shook my rattle around her body, the ancient way of sealing in the soul.

Miranda opened her eyes. She turned to me and I shared her soul retrieval.

"An eleven- going on twelve-year-old soul part showed up. She was running as fast as she could in a field."

"I remember that summer. My parents took me to Georgia to stay with a great aunt and uncle I'd never met. My parents were moving our family to a new house and thought I would be happier spending the summer in Georgia while they dealt with the move. I was their only child, so I was alone with these people I didn't know. I felt so uncomfortable there, not myself."

I beamed at her and said, "Welcome home."

•••••••••••••••••••

By the age of fifty, I was married with two children, licensed as a marriage, family, and child psychotherapist, and a certified practitioner in another therapeutic discipline called Body-Mind Centering, which explored movement, body (soma), and conscious awareness. That year I attended the annual conference of the Body-Mind Centering Association, which is where I met Annie Brook, who presented her work in healing birth trauma for children and adults. She was an appealing woman with a petite, muscular frame, a maternal smile, and shiny brown hair that swung around her jawline. I immediately felt I could trust her and was determined to get a firsthand experience with her. We arranged to meet in Colorado where she lived.

As I drove into Boulder, puffy white clouds spanned the horizon of the rich blue Colorado skies. Annie held her sessions in a round pool filled with body-temperature water. Together we were going to explore an old ache on the left side of my neck. I slid into the warm water, wearing my navy-blue one-piece suit. Breathing shallowly, I stood tucked against the edge, immersed up to my chin like an adolescent hiding at a pool party. Annie swam close and reached her arms toward me. My stomach fluttered as I grasped her open hands. *What will be revealed?* I knew that this process was deep, and that places I had never encountered in my twenty-five years as a therapist and healer would surface.

With Annie guiding me, I became a fish gliding along the surface of the water. "Follow my breath. Breathe in and out through your mouth," she instructed, while carefully placing a clip on my nose. "Now begin to imagine the sensations in utero, the tight, cushioned space." I folded my body in on itself and became as tiny as a human embryo.

Enveloped by Annie's arms, my Being remembered the in utero sensations. The pool water became amniotic fluid, and Annie's voice a distant guide. We moved as one, me inside her, inside my mother. There was nothing but pulsing heart and rhythmic breathing. An urgent desire to push came over me. Annie's arms became uterine walls, her legs a birth canal. I felt claustrophobic. *I'm* ready *to leave!*

Still curled in Annie's arms, below the surface now, my discomfort became profound. I struggled to uncurl the ball of my body. *Oh no!* I felt something stop me, constricting and angling my head. An evil cramp bit the left side of my neck. An electric shock poured through the narrow pathways from my heart to my head. I pushed my way to the surface, hauling Annie with me.

"I'm stuck . . . hard to breathe! There's a place right here in my heart so full of terror and death . . . and . . . I'm . . . blacking out!"

I draped myself over Annie's arms, and she held me as I inhaled for a moment, then she took me down into the darkness again. Down, down underwater, my eyes shut, the nose clip fastened tightly—down where all was still. Immovable. I froze, every cell gripping onto life. Nerves burned through my heart, and oxygen vanished inside me. Time was eternal. Right there I was taught stillness. Right there I learned to be between the worlds of life and death.

Carried by Annie, I floated on the current, dying. . . . The umbilical cord was wrapped around my neck. My soul, like a sharp sword, cut through, determined to live. The intense desire pulled me across the blackness.

Annie brought me up to the surface for air and intuited the experience I just had. "Slow yourself down now. Let the umbilical cord unravel around your neck." Every cell in my body heard this. *I am no longer dying.* My soul willed itself into my blood. I luxuriated in full, painless breaths of air filling my lungs. Breathing fully now, I was a little one ready for Life.

Annie sensed the shift and gently pulled me underwater again. My nerves had stopped burning. I swam with Annie, our bodies responding to each other as I squeezed through the birth canal, her powerful legs. Body and soul fused together, uniting in a force that was my birthright.

We surfaced. "I'm here. All of me," I whispered. Annie took me in her arms and cradled her freshly reborn.

PART TWO

CHAPTER FIVE

The Beginning

*In health the genial pretence must be kept up and the effort
renewed—to communicate, to civilise, to share, to cultivate
the desert, educate the native, to work together by day and by
night to sport. In illness this make-believe ceases. . . . We cease
to be soldiers in the army of the upright; we become deserters.*

— Virginia Woolf

I divorced in 2003, and in the fall of 2005, when Dana was a freshman and Cayla a junior in high school, we moved to a new house close to their school so we could participate in the social life of the community. I took down the garage and built a spacious dance studio complete with birch flooring, and began conducting private sessions for parents, infants, and children in my home studio. I used play to enhance motor development in ways that were therapeutic for the children and instructive for the parents.

Because Dana was going to India and Cayla to Ghana, Africa, for summer community service programs, we decided to host a fundraiser for the girls' trips. On a sweltering summer night, Dana, as master of ceremonies, flung open the doors to our studio, and our friends flocked in for the performances we'd lined up. We were all mesmerized and inspired by the musical expressions of our talented teenagers, but it was Cayla's dance performance that stood out.

Cayla made her way to the center of the stage and declared, "I want to end the evening with a traditional West African dance." Two classmates pounded the djembe drums open handed, starting in unison, then diverging into complex rhythms. Cayla's hair flew as her arms and legs beat out rhythm in the air. Her dance transported everyone out of the studio and into the African culture. It was a grand evening.

During this time in our lives, I would wake up every morning to the ever-present joy of endless possibilities. Our house was always full to the brim with friends, who would hang out for hours and often take the Kundalini Yoga classes I taught in the studio. Dana practiced her nature photography in the lush areas of our garden, and Cayla danced and painted. We were living my dream.

* * *

One day in January 2007, in the middle of Dana's sophomore year, while I was waiting in the pickup line at her school, my cell phone rang. I answered and Patrice, the mother of one of Dana's friends, informed me: "Your daughter brought over a water bottle full of vodka the other night before they went to the concert in Hollywood. She drank it and spent the evening in the alley throwing up."

"Really? I know she didn't have anything with her when I dropped her off." I remembered that Patrice's daughter, Nicole, had a reputation for drinking.

"Nicole said Dana brought the vodka. She was upset that she had to miss the concert to take care of Dana."

The car door opened and Dana got in.

"Thank you so much for calling, Patrice, I really appreciate it." I hung up.

"Was that Nicole's mom?"

"Yes. Apparently, you were pretty sick the other night."

She froze. I seized the stark quiet to say a few precious words.

"I expected you to experiment at this age, so here's my rule: If you are ever uncomfortable or in trouble, you call me, day or night, and I'll come get you. Make me the bad guy. Tell your friends I want you home, but never put yourself in danger. And I won't ask you about it."

Dana appeared stunned. I wasn't yelling at her or grounding her. I offered her support.

<hr/>

She never got a chance to call me. The following week on January 17, 2007, Dana came down with a fever overnight, followed by a knockdown fatigue. She became intolerably uncomfortable, and I didn't know what to do to help her. The illness manifested as a heavy cloak that wrapped itself around her. It became part of her skin and seeped inside her body. She felt pressure pounding in her head and a painful ache all over, as if the cloak had driven in nails. For her, the world got too loud, too complicated, too bright, full of unappealing smells as an almost inhuman hypersensitivity overtook her.

The pain, swelling, and fatigue became so severe that she had to quit school soon thereafter. She was out the entire second semester of tenth grade while doctors tried to diagnose her, and she would only leave the house for their appointments. She could not concentrate in conversation, read a book, or follow a movie. Anxiety and shortness of breath plagued her; however, the most difficult symptom was the pervasive swelling that expanded her body beyond its usual petite dimensions and made her feel less and less like herself. I bought her clothing in the next two sizes up from her normal size, because her swelling was unpredictable and she had to choose what clothes she could fit into on any given day. She had night sweats and chills during the day, even in the hottest weather.

Months went by. Everything slowed down as I watched the Dana I knew, the laughing, dancing athlete, disappear. She became a hypersensitive, angry teenager imprisoned in a personal hell, mindlessly staring at the TV. Her social life shrank as if it were a delicate garment thrown in the dryer by accident. The deterioration of her health, and the new, unwanted life that came with it, threatened both of us and called for a heroic patience neither of us yet knew we had.

In the beginning of Dana's illness, there were friends who stayed away, fearing she was contagious. She felt devastated. After the first week or two home from school, things began to go out of focus and continued to blur, sending us into survival mode for an unimaginable period of time. Dana was more and more isolated, crying daily, grieving and moaning about everything she missed.

A cloud of depression sat over our house, sucking up life. This silent desolation had no name, no warning, and no signposts. It caused a slow tsunami to crash over our family. Our life turned upside down. The worst thing was that nobody believed Dana was truly sick. Her own father, who had not lived with us for four years, imagined she was a severely depressed teen who needed psychiatric treatment. Even some of my friends accused me of spending too much time with her, of indulging her.

At the very beginning of Dana's illness, I took her to see Dr. Marcus, a respected integrative medicine doctor. He looked sweetly upon my sixteen-year-old daughter and said to me, "It's probably mono. I want to send her to the ear, nose, and throat doctor to confirm this." He checked her swollen lymph nodes, ordered lab tests, set up an appointment with the doctor across the hall, and gave her IV vitamin C to "perk her up."

Somewhat relieved, with labs in hand, we went to see Dr. Salberg, a balding, pasty, joyful man, who could moonlight as a stand-up comedian. When he met us in his office, he was wearing what looked like a miner's head lamp. He greeted us jovially, peered into Dana's facial orifices, and proclaimed, "She has the Epstein-Barr virus, which is a mononucleosis-like virus, and with rest, will be back to her old self in two months."

Approximately a month and a half later, when nothing had changed, Dr. Marcus sent Dana to Dr. Amara, an excellent infectious disease doctor, for more blood tests. Although the Epstein-Barr virus had shown up in her previous test and was thought to be the source of her endless fatigue, the new lab results showed nothing abnormal. Dr. Amara examined her and declared, "I know you don't feel well, but you're not swollen." She insinuated that Dana had some teenage need for attention. As we left the office, with tears streaming down her face, Dana wailed, "She thinks I'm making this up!"

With the new lab results, we returned to Dr. Marcus's office, where Dana was given B-vitamin injections and nutrients. He assured her, "You'll be as good as new in ten days!" (He, too, must have thought there was no real illness.) We were blindly hopeful again.

Over the next several months, our lives fell apart without a routine to our days. Dana lay in discomfort on the couch as our social life dwindled down to the twice weekly visits to Dr.

Marcus for her IV vitamin C. She lost everything dear to her sixteen-year-old self: hanging out with friends, going to school, afternoon dance classes, and simply getting out of the house. These losses, along with the fatigue, stomach pain, swelling, and headaches, made her depressed and resentful. Although Dr. Marcus had cheerfully promised Dana that she would be well in ten days, several more months passed and she was still terribly ill and debilitated.

* * *

"I will not give her antidepressants!" I stunned myself. Our lives changed in that one moment when I realized that Dana was not ailing from some kind of hormonally induced depression, nor was she suffering from any kind of common teen virus. Dreams began to burn up inside me; I had no place for this turn in our family road. I didn't have my bearings, but I was not going to be intimidated by Dr. Marcus.

Standing in front of him, staring into his critical face, I was aghast at his attempt to humiliate me into giving Dana antidepressants. Dr. Marcus was frustrated that she wasn't progressing and bellowed at me, "Would you not give your daughter insulin if she were diabetic?" I looked in his eyes, and in that moment, lost faith in him. I stood there feeling empty as I stared into his strained face and wondered if I was strong enough to take Dana's illness into my own hands.

I demanded, "What's wrong with her gut?"

Silence. I left without the prescriptions, fired him in my mind, and set out to help my daughter, no matter what it would take. We walked out the giant glass doors, leaving behind all the doctors with no answers. I put my arm around Dana's shoulders, and we entered the void together, a mother-daughter duet, fueled by my desire to piece our lives back together and prevent her from further suffering. She cried softly, the achy muscles and pounding head walking out the doors with us. "I'm going to figure out how to get you better!"

Within a month my life came to a standstill, and I retreated inside myself. It was the only way I could keep myself sane while taking care of Dana. Her moans and screams tore through my nerves like shards of glass. I stopped scheduling regular sessions for clients and stopped teaching yoga. I hovered over my daughter, her sole caretaker and medical advocate. I sent the seventy-five pages of lab results to more specialists, infectious disease doctors, and rheumatologists, which only resulted in being able to rule out more conditions. I was determined to find the source of Dana's illness. I couldn't stop. She would not be sentenced to a life of pain, and I would not be sentenced to a life of misery.

• • • • • • • • • • ⁕ • • • • • • • • • •

After the failure with Dr. Marcus, I took Dana to see a Chinese herbalist who had had success with conditions undiagnosed by medical doctors. He checked her acupuncture points and formulated special herbs, convinced she was suffering from toxic mold. *Mold!* I ripped my house apart looking for damp spots. This frightened me for weeks; I felt responsible for her pain. I hired a mold inspection company, removed panels off the exterior siding, and put moisture collectors in every room. In Dana's room I saw something suspicious—a tiny spot of mold on the wooden floor right in front of her bed! Unbeknownst to me, a sprinkler had been spraying an insignificant stream of water into the screened opening in the crawl space just under Dana's room. I panicked and moved her into the guest room while I had the floor repaired.

After nine months of illness, we suspected it was more than mold. Dana had made no improvement. We tested her for heavy metal toxicity and discovered high levels of arsenic. Another hidden danger! The previous summer she had spent five weeks in a rural village in India working on her community service project. I did some internet research and learned that arsenic had been found in India's groundwater. I read a list of dangerous symptoms; she had three: headaches, confusion, and drowsiness. Dana began a chelating treatment, intended to remove heavy metals from the body, which lasted three months, and then a parasite cleanse, which made her feel worse. As a part of this whole treatment, she also took supplements and applied a stinky cream to her belly every day to draw out the arsenic. Three months later her arsenic levels were down, but she was no better.

In addition to her other symptoms, Dana was experiencing a mysterious nervous system imbalance and agitation at night. She couldn't fall asleep before the wee hours of the morning. One day she fell asleep during the afternoon. This nap lasted more than three hours, and I became terrified that she would never wake up. I tiptoed into her room and soundlessly put my ear next to her nose to listen for her breathing. All was quiet except the whisper of her breath. I knew in that instant what it might feel like for the umbilical lifeline from mother to daughter to be severed. These thoughts shivered through me as I imagined the hum of her sweet spirit missing in my life.

On occasion Dana would spend the whole day in her room laboriously preparing to go to a punk rock concert much later that night. She would have to rest in between showering and putting her clothes on, but she was hell-bent on getting out of the house. She would appear before me dressed from head to toe in black and demand that I drive her to the concert. My hope that she was somehow getting better would cloud my judgment. I couldn't say no to her. I would drive her to a punk rock music club called the Echo, a good hour or more from our house, let her out in front, park, and wait for her text letting me know she was ready to leave.

Nevertheless, no matter what I did for her, she was always bitter or angry with me. One day when she was again listlessly lying on the couch, I found myself hissing at her, "Now that you're home all day, you must at least do your own dishes—and try to go outside once in a while."

Dana snapped, "Stop yelling at me."

"I'm not yelling," I said through clenched teeth. With that, I turned away from her and walked very deliberately into the kitchen, my refuge. *What's happening to us?*

I marched back into the living room and declared, "You have to get on with your life somehow! This is so fucking hard!"

Silence. Lots of silence. I knew I'd gone too far. But I was worn out, confused, and desperate. I was convinced that some of her behavior, her anger and listlessness, had to be a symptom of teenage rebellion.

Dana bolted from the couch and ran down the hall, tortured by the purgatory of her damaged existence. She flew into her room. I sped after her and caught the bronze handle of her door just as she slammed it in my face. I held on to it so she couldn't lock it. I was fuming as I stared at the white-paneled door, feeling her grip on the other side. In that moment I yelled louder than I ever have in all my years of parenting. "You can handle my anger, you're strong. If you come out in three minutes and face me, I'll have deep respect for you." I waited for what felt like years.

The door flew open with only thirty seconds to spare. I loved her in that moment even more than I hurt.

I grabbed her hand and said, "Come with me. I want you to hear something." I dragged her to the stereo in the living room. I inserted a CD and said, "Listen."

Her girlfriend Savannah's poignant, melodic song filled the air between us.

"All I want for you, is to be free. . . . What I want for you, is to live endlessly. . . . All I want for you, is to be healed. . . . What I want to give you is a sword and shield, and know that all I want for you, is to finally feel alive."

Tears rolled down my cheeks as the lyrics expressed what I had not managed to say to Dana. We were in a terrible struggle. She was fighting for the independence she was rightfully due, and I was fighting for her life.

In September 2007 Dana was finally able to return to school part-time for eleventh grade. Unable to dance, which had been an expressive outlet for her, she began taking voice lessons. Richard, her voice teacher, would come to our house and accompany Dana on our piano as she sang like a rock star, exorcising her anger and pain. I too began to sing again, enjoying the thrill of my own voice as I polished off the entire *Yentl* songbook.

Eventually Dana's breathing became too laborious to continue singing, so poetry surfaced as her new mode of expression. Patti Smith and the bold, subversive women of the punk era spoke with enough fire and brilliance to inspire Dana's inner voice. She took up writing with ferocity and dedication, and produced a poem that spoke to her pain and frustration:

The Secrets of a Seashell
Poisonous snakes slithering in my muscles
And rattling their tails in my blood-pooled joints,
Expanded blowfish seeping out of my fragile skull,
Sharp-toothed piranhas swimming expectantly in my belly,
A robe of stones invisibly swathing my weak body.

"Something is wrong," I say!
The white-cloaked men tell me this isn't so.
"I have a wild imagination," they say,
"Take these chemicals and this will 'go away.'"

The blowfish get angry,
The piranhas and snakes get violent,
White-cloaked man after white-cloaked man conclude
That I cannot be fixed,
That it is the fault of my own.

"Keep at it," I say to myself,
"I think I would know if I was the cause of such treachery."
I will not cost my determination its goal for
what someone else has said.
I must keep my mind still, inside a sterile glass case.
It is only with a pure mind that we can truly succeed.

I breathe in peace each day to calm the deadly beasts
that I am temporarily housing.
In the end I shall win,
In the end I will smile because I will prove to
the white-cloaked world that I was right,
That I am not alone.

They have not been listening sweetly enough
To the seashell to hear the sound of the ocean.
They will see, soon enough they will see.
They will shiver in their own ice-castles of remorse!

CHAPTER SIX

Road Trip

Nothing behind me, everything ahead of me,
as is ever so on the road.

— Jack Kerouac

By the second semester of her junior year, Dana was struggling with symptoms that mirrored nervous system conditions: agitation and sleep problems. From the beginning she had experienced swelling, fatigue, and body pain, but more symptoms kept developing. It was never the same from day to day—some days were better, some days worse. I had become deeply concerned as the agitation and sleeplessness grew worse. Precious time ticked away while something attacked my daughter. There was a madwoman inside me running stark naked down the middle of the street, screaming for help.

I had to take action. I was terrified of brain damage after reading about nervous system disorders, ready to try anything and everything. Around this time I ran into Cheryl, an old friend and health practitioner, who recommended we try the Life Vessel, a device developed to balance the autonomic nervous system, increase lymphatic drainage, and detoxify the body.

During Dana's spring break, we flew to Santa Fe for the first in what would become a series of treatments with the Life Vessel at an alternative health clinic, hoping they would resolve her difficulty sleeping, relieve her pain, and calm her anxiety. Once there, a diagnostic test of her autonomic nervous system revealed that she was indeed agitated and had difficulty calming down. The Life Vessel, an elegantly crafted, large coffin-shaped box, is where Dana rested for her first hour-long treatment. Joanne, the owner of the clinic, made sure she was comfortable and warm, then closed the lid on the box and started the treatment. Inside, a star formation of lights in primary colors flashed above her eyes, and gorgeous classical music filled the space with sound as the foam bed on which she lay vibrated. Joanne explained that this system was designed to utilize sensory stimuli to engage the body systems for the purpose of healing disease.

I sat reading and praying in the waiting room. I prayed that these Life Vessel sessions would transform Dana back into a normal teen. I visualized her strong legs running on the track at school, or jazz dancing in our studio at home. I saw her tumbling gracefully through gravity on aerial silk. I peered over her shoulder as she finished her homework at the kitchen table, and I listened while she gossiped and laughed with friends.

When we returned home after Dana completed the treatment, she was too weak to go back to school. Joanne had told us she would need several series of treatments in order to "turn the corner." Our lives had been stuffed into the pocket of a discarded garment. Dana lay on the couch in excruciating discomfort while her classmates went to the Spring Prom and finished their junior year, so I decided to schedule a second series of treatments for her a month later. Exasperated with her isolation, and furious that she wouldn't be moving on to the senior year with her class, Dana insisted in a bloodthirsty voice that I *drive* her to Santa Fe for the next treatments.

"I'm going completely crazy! All I do is sit on the couch while my friends are enjoying their lives. I have to get out of here! I'm sick of staring at the four walls of the living room. I will die if I don't have a change of scenery!"

She was desperate for anything to distract her from the loneliness, pain, and agitation she felt. I needed time to think about this. How could I risk taking her out of the house in her condition? What mother would take her sick child on a road trip through the desert? In spite of my fears, it didn't take long to make my decision. It was clear to me that I had to do something to keep Dana from despair, so I amassed maps and calculated distances between places of interest in California, Arizona, Utah, Colorado, and New Mexico. I began to get excited! The vision of Thelma and Louise became our inspiration. We were getting out of town, breaking the rules, checking out of our daily lives at home, being impulsive, and defying the debilitating illness that gave us no vacation. We were rebels following Dana's intuitive calling. Really, we were two women in a blue Lexus wagon piled high with food rations, pots, hot plates, silverware, dishes, a blender, pillows, clothes, alkaline water, and an oil diffuser—all the essentials. We were bound for adventure!

We drove out of Los Angeles at sundown so there wouldn't be any sunlight to irritate Dana's sensitive eyes—a troubling new symptom. Five hours later we stopped in Kingman, Arizona, at the Holiday Inn Express, where the lobby smelled like Pine Sol. I piled everything packed in our car onto the rickety baggage cart, including bags of Chinese foot patches—two-by-three-inch adhesive rectangles infused with zeolite for drawing out toxins. I snuck through the hallway to our room, barely controlling the cart. I moved us in, unpacked, made Dana's bed with the fresh sheets we brought, and began cooking dinner: quinoa and vegetables prepared on our own hot plate. I prepared food that had been prescribed for the alkaline cleanse diet she had recently adopted. The cleanse was meant to create enough alkalinity in her system to kill off any microorganisms that might be causing her illness.

We woke at noon. Dana took out her camera and immortalized me bending over the cart making myself an almond butter sandwich for the road. She thought it was funny, but I knew I had to be prepared. I had to make sure I ate enough before we headed out because I couldn't stop the car along the road if Dana was asleep for fear of waking her to her discomfort. She always felt uncomfortable and sleep offered a respite. "Mom, just keep driving, don't stop. I need to see the scenery go by. I need to be distracted from the pain." After I loaded the car and Dana applied the two Chinese patches on each foot, we headed toward the Grand Canyon.

At an overlook, we took in the cavernous cleavage in the earth, marveling at the layers of rusts and golds flaming in the sunlight. Dana and I moved gingerly down a path, admiring the canyon's majesty. I did not know then that this would be one of only a handful of times she would be able to get out of the car to see the sights on our trip.

Years ago my father had joyously taken me, my sisters, and my mother to see every geyser, paint pot, and thermal spring in Yellowstone National Park. After that trip, he took us camping on weekends and vacations to as many state and national parks as we could drive to in our blue Ford station wagon. He built a wooden box and strapped it to the top of the car to store our camping gear, old hiking clothes, and frying pans. My father wanted to show us as much of the world as he could, driving us as far east as Wyoming, as far south as Mexico City, and as far north as Vancouver.

In this moment I became my father and enthusiastically took Dana around the entire perimeter of the south rim, with drive-by close-ups of every scenic viewpoint. She leaned out the window with her camera shutter flapping. It began to hail as we stopped at a scenic lookout. I ran outside to gaze at the view and hurried back to the car. "Dana! You have to come see this!" As I helped her out, we were pelted by tiny frozen snowballs. The light was ethereal at sunset in the hail, and we were both awed by the dramatic vista of blue sky and dark clouds over a vivid palette of earthen colors. Caught in a moment of freedom and shocking beauty, we doubled over, laughing as hard as the wind blew. Dana, enveloped in swirling white specks, raincoat billowing wildly, stole my heart with her smile.

Leaving the park as the sun fell, we continued to follow the rim's perimeter until the road dove lower and lower into the desert terrain. I had a lot on my shoulders—everything actually. I was responsible for making sure we had all the necessities for our survival in remote areas. Dana had become hypersensitive to temperature, sound, light, and smell, so I did whatever I could to accommodate her. This was a difficult way to live, and on the road I had less control over the environment than I did at home. As a consequence, Dana sat beside me whimpering. After all the stimulation of the day, her head throbbed and she couldn't bear to talk anymore.

A few hours later we pulled into our motel in the tiny suburban town of Page at Lake Powell. I did the drill with the cart, through the lobby to our room, trying not to knock into walls or send things flying. I slept, deprived and exhausted from performing the job of driver, cook, caretaker, nose wiper, emotional cheerleader, and environmental controller. That night Dana's body went into high gear as usual, racing like a car in park with the gas pedal pressed all the way down.

"Momma, will you stay with me?"

"Of course, honey."

It was impossible for her to fall asleep until exhaustion knocked her out around three or four in the morning.

The next day we wound lazily through the picturesque formations of Lake Powell. We stopped and I encouraged Dana to get out of the car. "I couldn't help but stop here—it's so extraordinary. Will you stand at the top of that sandy ridge so I can take your picture?" She smiled; it was early in the day. She crawled out of the car and hobbled to the top of the ridge. I captured her standing with her feet apart and her arms flying up in a "V for victory," high above the turquoise lake in the background. In defiance of her illness, Dana's cheeks pinked and her eyes gleamed with triumph.

We left the lake, heading west, driving along the lower edge of southern Utah. Hours of spectacular scenery passed by as we listened to the calm, nurturing voice of Jack Kornfield narrating his audio book *The Roots of Buddhist Psychology*. We were inspired by the Buddhist mindset, listening to Jack's voice calmly mentoring us as a father might kindly mentor a child. He spoke of one's interior life and what brought awakening, freedom, and happiness. Jack taught us that one needs skills to still the mind.

"Momma, let's leave our fears behind and soak up the land in Utah with mindfulness and joy!" It appeased my fear to hear Dana say that; however, inside me was a mother in tattered clothing, worn out and sleep deprived.

Being with Dana was blissful at times. It felt like we were bonding in ways most mothers and daughters never do. It was a silent rhythm of glory and guts. Our hearts grew warmer in each other's presence, and we shared a vast fear no one else could grasp. We held on to each other against the world.

Other times we were faced with the tension of discomfort, fear, and discord.

"Stop making that chewing noise, Mom. I can't stand the smell of your sandwich." I kept quiet, pulling in my frustration.

Everything bothered Dana. When pain overwhelmed her ability to be civil, we drove in silence. It was during these daytime drives that she soothed herself from the discomfort of bloating and headaches by wearing a device called the Microcurrent. This was a small battery-operated box that used mild electrical currents to reduce inflammation in the body, balance the adrenals, stimulate parts of the brain, and stabilize moods. To use this device, Dana attached probes that connected the box to the front and back of her body. These probes were wrapped in small, damp terry cloth towels to conduct the electrical current. She also wrapped a moist hand towel around her neck and one around her feet to guide the current through her whole body. She was embarrassed to be seen like this and hunkered down in her seat to hide if I stopped for gas or food. The irony was that no one was around for miles and miles.

We drove through large sandstone canyon walls into Zion National Park. At one point the road tunneled right through the stately, auburn rock. We were speechless for miles. As the sun drifted down, the changing light illuminated shiny, bronze boulders on all sides, hues of melting rust washed over them. There was something larger than us, larger than our fears, confusion, or even Dana's physical pain. This road trip served a purpose, guiding us somehow. Nothing was more precious than being this close to each other. I looked over at Dana's face and saw something I hadn't seen before. She reached her hand out to mine with a sober grasp.

As the third day drew to a close, we checked into a motel in St. George, Utah. Because the nights were so difficult, we'd brought a variety of things to help Dana sleep: soothing CDs, homeopathic remedies, and essential oils. Up at noon, we scurried to eat, shower, and pack up the car. The routine was seamless. I knew exactly where to stash the bags, gear, and food, and had it down to twenty minutes, tops. I felt the promise of a new day! Dana was sitting in the passenger seat with the key in the ignition and the power turned on, listening to her iPod, while I loaded the car. Ready to go, I glided into the driver's seat, turned the key, and heard a dull grind. It wasn't the gas— the tank was full. I tried again. It was dead. The battery. Sucked dry by the iPod.

I glanced over at Dana. "Unplug your iPod. I'm going inside the hotel for some help."

On my way back I paused by the side of the building, out of Dana's sight. I wanted to scream at her, but it wasn't her fault. She didn't know her iPod would drain the battery. She didn't know I was at my breaking point. I wanted to belt out, "STOP THIS!" I pushed against the beige stucco wall with both fists, imagining what it would feel like to pound them into a bloody pulp. I pushed harder. I had been thrown into a lion's den, my life ripped from me as fangs sliced through flesh. I kicked the wall, hard. It hurt. I held back the tears that had been welling up all morning. *STOP THIS, God dammit!*

I was shaking inside. Everything turned to fear. Before the trip I was worried about whether I would have the stamina to drive the long distances and take care of Dana. But now, for the first time, I faced the risk I'd taken by driving on remote, backcountry roads with a sick daughter. *Will the battery go out again? Will we be in the middle of nowhere?* I had the car thoroughly inspected before we left LA, but out here we were alone. *Alone.* I would be alone with a sick daughter, far from a doctor of any kind. The beige stucco wall came into sharp focus as I looked up. I stopped myself, wrenching my mind back to center. I took a deep breath. With conviction I bravely decided to have faith until a real dilemma presented itself.

I returned to the car. With as much equanimity as I could muster, I turned to Dana and said sweetly, "We'll just sit tight for a few minutes until the maintenance man can come give us a jump."

"I didn't do it on purpose. I'm sorry, Mom." My insides melted.

An hour later we set out for the interior of Utah, headed toward the ancient rocks of Bryce Canyon. Dana plugged her iPod in and was content for the ride. I meditated on the car battery holding up. We never had another problem with it. Grand, castle-like stone pillar formations rose up on either side of the highway, forming a gateway. I grabbed a park brochure at the entrance and pulled over to see where to go.

"Dana, it says here the formations are called 'hoodoos.'"

"Who knew?" She giggled.

They looked like Disney creations. Nature was complex and astonishing.

"It says here, 'The earth's crust rose and fell over centuries, and weather patterns sculpted the many layers of varied rock and sand.'"

It comforted me to feel insignificant in the face of this grandeur. Our jaws dropped as we ventured farther into the park. At a canyon overlook we peered down into the valley and saw a stone fortress with thousands of hoodoo "soldiers" standing at attention. A mesmerizing sight. We sat under a tree at the cliff's edge until the sun dipped down and were treated to a stunning show of the last light over the captivating soldiers. As I looked more closely, I saw the outline of each soldier, an army of individuals.

We secured the only room for miles around so we could stay another day. I unlocked the door and wilted at the sight of the garage sale décor.

"Momma, just look at this quaint place, it's so adorable! Not anything like the generic rooms we've been staying in!"

"So glad you like it here, sweetheart! I'll try to spice up your quinoa and veggies tonight too."

Enlivened by the majesty of Bryce Canyon and the quirky motel room, Dana picked up one of the books she'd brought and started reading it out loud to me. With tears in my eyes, I listened as she read the first chapter of *On the Road*. This was the first time in a year that she'd had the ability to focus her attention enough to read. Her voice was tinny and wobbly, but she kept on reading. "The only people for me are the mad ones, the ones who are mad to live, mad to talk, mad to be saved." *Clearly we are Kerouac's mad ones!*

The next day we drove into the tiny town of Teasdale, Utah, where we found lodgings in an unexpectedly charming cabin. The property was surrounded by dark red rocks rising in towerlike formations that obscured the flat, desert terrain. They loomed all around, creating a walled-city effect. We nourished ourselves with a two-night stay and woke the first day to the sight of hot, red boulders flaming in the sun, as seen through our bay windows. We enjoyed a day without driving. I hiked some, Dana rested and drew. My cell phone rang while I was perched atop a large boulder. I listened to Dr. Morgan, an integrative doctor from the Life Vessel clinic, relay the results of a recent blood test. Not enough protein. Oh God, maybe that was the root of the problem! Dana had taken it upon herself to become a vegetarian when she was in middle school because she felt bad about killing animals. Had she compromised her health by not getting enough animal fat and protein?

"Dana, Dr. Morgan said your test shows a lack of protein." I knew she might balk.

"Does this mean I have to eat meat?"

"Let's start with some fish tonight."

"Okay, Momma. I'll do it if you think it will help."

A day later we were on the road again with hours of dry land, low mountains, and no civilization. It was as Louise said on the road trip with Thelma: "Well, we're not in the middle of nowhere, but we can see it from here." I tasted dirt and felt grit between my teeth. We finally arrived in Hanksville. Actually we drove past it, hypnotized by hot, flat lands and endless, straight roads. We'd been told about Hanksville by a man in the only gift shop in Teasdale, who said, "It's the best rock shop in all of Utah."

We pulled up in front of an old, dusty sign saying "Rock Shop," with piles of rocks in rusty bins flanking the front. On our way in we were greeted by an old woman, thoroughly wrinkled by age and sun. She apologized for the fact that the legendary proprietor, Ernie Shirley, had recently died at age ninety. Ernie's prized, giant dinosaur bone, one of the greatest fossil specimens ever found, lay on the ground out in the back. The story goes that after finding it in the wild country surrounding Hanksville, he loaded it onto a wheelbarrow, rolled it for miles over the rocky desert terrain, lowered it down a sheer cliff, and brought it home intact.

"Hey, Dana, look at this bin of petrified dino poop! They're so pretty. Who can we get one of these for?"

Dana's face cracked open. "How about Cayla?" She cackled.

Twenty minutes north of Hanksville, Goblin Valley turned out to be eleven worthwhile miles off the San Rafael Desert's main road. We cruised through low hills and shrubs, keeping our eyes on a single monolithic rock in the distance. The road slimmed down to barely one lane before we reached the Goblin Valley State Park. The "goblins" are mushroom-shaped formations up to twenty feet high that give the illusion of creatures. These formations have large orange-brown boulders of hard rock that look like heads, with weaker sandy layers underneath eroded into thinner bodies. Over millions of years, wind and rain carved the goblins in groups. They appeared lifelike and eerie surrounded by the vast desert. Dana stayed in the car, and I walked up close to the goblins, the only person in the walled valley.

We left the goblins and headed north. Once again there was nothing but the straight road through low desert brush, with occasional sculpted stone pinnacles to attract my attention. At this point we were listening to the Jack Kornfield CD for the second time: "When we let go of our battles and open our heart to things as they are, then we come to rest in the present moment. . . . Only in this moment can we discover that which is timeless." Dana dozed while I breathed in these words.

We hit the main highway and headed to Arches National Park, six miles north of Moab, Utah. In town we found a health food store with local organic produce. Dana was so excited, we stayed two nights. We spent the following day exploring Arches. The park was home to over two thousand natural sandstone arches, hundreds of soaring pinnacles, massive fins, and giant balanced rocks. Driving into the monumental 76,518-acre park, we gazed at formations with names such as "Balanced Rock," "Delicate Arch," and "Broken Arch." The landscape was eye-opening. Mountains gave way to deep canyons and vast mesas hung over broad valleys of red desert. We drove to a cliff-edge viewpoint, thinking this might be the place where Thelma and Louise drove off in the last scene of the film.

"Dana, can you spot the Thunderbird Louise drove off the cliff here?"

"Nope."

"Just as well. We're different, you and me. We're bound for life!"

We left Moab, driving out of Utah into Colorado. The scenery turned greener as we cruised through low mountains dotted with shrubs that eventually gave way to dense pine forests and rivers. When we arrived in Telluride, we rented a condo for two nights at the Mountain Lodge, the essence of rustic elegance. We were on the fourth floor in a room with views of the newest green grass I'd ever seen, laid out over rolling hills decorated with tall pines in the distance. We each had our own bedroom, which was heaven for me. I'm not a complainer, but I rarely had a break from Dana's discomfort. Just lying on the bed staring out the window elevated me. After helping Dana get to sleep, I was free to relax in my room with a romance novel. The simple plotlines and the predictable endings gave me comfort.

Dana was having a better day, so we took the gondola down the mountain to explore the town of Telluride in the valley below our lodge. We poked around the tourist shops and ended up buying Dana a blue sundress with a delicate lace neckline and embroidered bodice. She changed into it right away, thrilled with how feminine and pretty she looked in the mirror. Her eyes widened, color filled her face, and little tears formed on her lower lids.

"I feel good in this dress, Momma."

This was a special day. Dana was feeling well enough to go out to a restaurant for dinner. There were white table-cloths, fine wines, and well-dressed patrons. Our salmon arrived perfectly seared, with little rose potatoes and julienned carrots on the side. A mountain of crispy, tangled onions dressed the salmon. I was transported to another time when dining had been a pleasure and we had occasions to celebrate. Dana enjoyed everything, including our conversation. This *was* a vacation! We sipped tea after the meal and luxuriated in the moment. On the way back to the gondola, in the street by the curb, Dana released her entire meal, soiling the hem of her new, blue dress. I was devastated. It took all my strength to navigate her weak body into the gondola and back to our room.

Durango was our last stop before we reached Santa Fe. Here we rented a little two-bedroom log cabin by a lake. We cooked and rested and sat outside under a large tree canopy, talking. Dana had finished *On the Road* and began to read out loud from Noah Levine's book, *Against the Stream: A Buddhist Manual for Spiritual Revolutionaries.* Dana knew Noah from attending his Buddhist meditation Dharma Punx group in Hollywood. She and I talked about the story of his recovery, which led him to a Buddhist practice of forgiveness and allowed him to recognize the interconnectedness of all things. In his book he recounts a year of meditating on his own death. In Buddhist practice, one must see the world as it actually is. Pain exists, but suffering is a function of the mind.

Two sunny days later, we were back in the car, driving toward Santa Fe. We arrived and unloaded at the Sage Inn for the week. The Life Vessel treatments started the following day.

After four days of lying in the humming, vibrating, pulsating coffin, Dana was still tired, swollen, and headachy. In the hotel at night, I gently used my hands to soothe her head.

"I'm going to help your cranial-sacral fluids to flow through the system." I held her head in my hands at the base of her cranial bones, supporting her neck. "How does this feel, Dana?"

"It's helping. But it feels like a big fat stupid depressed man, sometimes angry, is in my head, and his fat is seeping through the holes in my skull."

I could feel through my hands the tightness releasing and the rhythm of the cranial fluids becoming stronger. It would only be effective for about fifteen minutes. Dana's "big fat stupid depressed man" would undo my gentle healing.

Joanne went out of her way to provide for Dana's improvement. She asked us if we would stay two extra days so Dana could pose as the "patient" in a demonstration of a new treatment the clinic was considering. This new treatment was invented by a military vet named Bud, who'd healed his own injured body by using high-powered magnets. He developed a way to use a 150-pound, torso-shaped magnet plate for healing. Impatient for something new to relieve Dana's swelling and pain, we decided to stay. Bud asked her to lie on the magnet for twenty minutes. The first ten minutes she lay on her belly, and the last ten on her back. I went in with Bud to see her at the end. I glanced down at her legs and began to weep. I hadn't seen her kneecaps in over a year. Clearly, this magnet was helping. It allowed the lymphatic system to function at its best. I didn't understand how, but I could see the results. Bud had an extra one for sale; we bought it on the spot and loaded it into the back of my Lexus where Dana could lie on it while we traveled. This heavy, handmade device changed her life. We hauled the magnet around for the next four years; it was the *only* thing that gave Dana relief from ongoing swelling.

On the way home we stopped in Sedona for the night. I carried everything into the hotel room, leaving the magnet in the car. By the time we got up at midday, it was blisteringly hot, over one hundred degrees. I could cook a pot of quinoa on the magnet! I covered it with hotel towels and parked the car under a shade tree, leaving the back hatch open so Dana could lie on it again before we got back on the road. I checked on her several times to make sure she hadn't passed out from the heat.

Late in the afternoon, we headed back to Los Angeles, driving through the desert moonscape of Arizona and California, arriving in Northridge after midnight. We were home from our risky adventure, wiped out but hopeful that our new magnet plate would cure her swelling.

CHAPTER SEVEN

Positive

*Our own sorrows seem heavy enough, even when
lifted by certain long-term joys. But watching others
hurt is the breaker of most any heart.*

— Clarissa Pinkola Estés

In July 2008, a month after we returned from the Santa Fe
clinic, Dana and I were planning to go to Northampton,
Massachusetts, where I would assist the teacher in the Infant
Developmental Movement course at the school where I'd
received my training in this somatic discipline. My practice had
been impacted by the unpredictable nature of Dana's illness,
but I loved my work.

The night before we were to leave, a crisis occurred. We
placed the magnet plate on a massage table in the room next
to Dana's bedroom. Since the magnet plate was relatively new
to us, we'd been experimenting by increasing the amount of
time Dana would lie on it from thirty minutes to one hour. At

bedtime she positioned herself on the plate and said, "I've set the timer, Mom, so you don't have to come in to get me. I'll be able to make it to bed on my own."

I heard the timer beeping from my bedroom but decided to wait for half an hour before I looked in on Dana. I'd been hovering, which irritated her, so I gave her the space to take care of herself. When I finally went in to check on her, she was still lying on the plate. She'd fallen asleep and had been lying on the magnet for well over an hour. I gently helped her off the massage table and into bed. At about 2:30 a.m. I woke up to her fragile voice crying, "Mommy."

I bolted into Dana's room and found her shivering in a fetal position. "I can't move, and I can't get warm," she moaned. She was so weak I was worried she would die in front of me. I split into two: part of me took action and spoke softly and lovingly to her; the other part froze.

"I never fell back to sleep, Mom," Dana whispered to me. I ran to get down feather blankets. Then I called the "magnet man."

"Bud, so sorry to call in the middle of the night, but I don't know what to do and I need your help. Dana's shivering and can't move. This happened after she spent over an hour on the magnet."

"Okay, get her warm. Give her hot tea and put her into the sauna until her body can warm itself. Anna, stay calm and let me know what happens."

Bud had no idea what bodily system, organ, or gland had been thrown off by the magnet, causing the frigid shutdown, but he explained that we had to work up to one hour more slowly.

I got in the sauna with Dana, turned it up to high, and sat in my sweaty pajamas waiting for her to come to life again.

After twenty minutes she lifted her head and said clearly, "Mom, I'm ready to get out. I'm warm enough."

I took her back to her room and fell asleep with her. In the early morning before dawn, I woke before she did and felt a calm settling over me, knowing we won the fight for another day. I sat awake wondering what the daylight would bring. I knew I had to cancel our trip.

When Dana woke up, she surprised me by saying, "I want to stick with our plan, but can we leave a day later so I can regain my strength?" I trusted her instincts, and I wanted to go—badly. This was my opportunity to collaborate with colleagues. "Okay, I'll change our flights."

We checked into a lovely old farmhouse where the owner, Carol, raised flowers and butterflies. Built in the 1700s, the farmhouse featured two bedrooms, a small living room–library, a bathroom, and a little eat-in kitchen with windows facing the garden. Dana was charmed. Though I hoped the peaceful surroundings would be healing for her, I thought I smelled mold, and probably did. Nonetheless, I said nothing to Dana and instead pulled out my arsenal of essential oils and filled the diffuser with oils that would purify the air.

Dana's bedroom had a raised platform where the bed stood, and above on the low dormer ceiling hung large, blown-up photographs of cocoons drooping from branches in varying stages of development. The cocoons looked like fibrous, fluorescent light conductors with moist chrysalises inside. The photos of butterflies just beginning to emerge from their cocoons revealed a secret moment. Dana woke every morning to these images, working their way into her psyche.

Since we couldn't travel with the 150-pound magnet plate, Dana slept on a thirty-pound magnet mattress pad that Bud sent to us. He explained that she could lie on the pad for six hours at a time because it was far less powerful than the plate. I set my alarm for six hours, got up when it beeped, and quietly crept into Dana's room to slip the pad out from under her. A metallic smell always lingered in the air after she woke up, so we used a room diffuser with essential oils to clean the air and help with the odor from her detoxing body. We figured she was detoxing heavy metals through her skin.

The magnet mattress pad had been designed to kill pathogens, unlike the magnet plate, which was designed specifically to detoxify the body by stimulating lymphatic drainage. The magnetic field of the small magnets in the pad penetrated about two inches into the body, making it difficult for most pathogens to survive.

We happened to be staying smack-dab in the middle of Lyme tick country, and one night, after I brushed a dark speck from my neck, I called Carol, frantic for her to help me figure out if I had a tick bite. She brought a chart showing the tick development cycle and what to look for. We spent at least two hours worrying about whether or not I might have been bitten by a tick carrying Lyme disease. The irony was that we still had no idea that Dana was suffering from what we would soon learn was *full-blown* chronic Lyme disease.

Back home I researched Lyme disease because I was concerned about myself, and I discovered that I didn't have the symptoms but Dana did. In an effort to understand the disease, I spoke to a woman who'd had it for many years. She explained to me that the standard Lyme tests often produce false negative results and recommended getting a blood test at the lab Lyme doctors use. I had Dr. Morgan from the Life Vessel clinic write the order for this blood test.

I walked out to the miniature replica of our house that was our mailbox to check the mail for the third day in a row. There in the pile was a large envelope from the lab! I ripped it open, praying for an answer to our agony. My eyes followed the printed words next to the Western blot test. I felt weightless, as if I were sitting at the top of a Ferris wheel before it plunged downward. P-O-S-I-T-I-V-E for Lyme disease! Holy shit! There it was on paper, the diagnosis previous tests denied.

Suppressing the growing hysteria in my voice, I called out as I entered the house: "Dana, your test came back positive! I've got to get you to a Lyme doctor! Oh my God!"

My spine throbbed with holy terror as I remembered the frightening things I'd heard about Lyme. I knew it was a bad disease. I became confused. *Should I be elated or devastated that we finally had a diagnosis?* I prayed that now Dana could get the right treatment—if it wasn't too late.

Looking back, there were little clues all along. In 2004, when Dana was thirteen years old, she was diagnosed with morphea (a rare skin condition) on her leg, which we later found out is an autoimmune response often resulting from Lyme infection. That was the most obvious visible clue. She also suffered from stomach bloating and swollen legs, as well as severe headaches and digestive discomfort, in the year before she became completely debilitated by illness. After incorrect diagnoses of fibromyalgia, chronic fatigue syndrome, heavy metal toxicity, and clinical depression, we had finally discovered the root cause of her systemic symptoms.

Dana's symptoms now included persistent swollen glands, sore throat, fevers, joint issues (pain, stiffness, swelling), muscle issues (pain, weakness, cramps), mental issues (confusion, difficulty thinking and concentrating, problems absorbing new information, forgetfulness, poor short-term memory, poor attention), emotional issues (mood swings, irritability, depression, anxiety, panic attacks), headaches, light and sound sensitivity, eye floaters, unstable balance, light-headedness, neck stiffness, neck pain, fatigue, poor stamina, sleep issues (insomnia, fractionated sleep, early awakening), unexplained menstrual irregularity, stomach and abdominal issues (queasy stomach, nausea, stomach pain, digestive discomfort, low abdominal pain, cramps), heart palpitations, chest wall pain, head congestion, breathlessness, and night sweats.

I was able to get Dana an appointment to see Dr. Farber, a well-respected "Lyme Literate" doctor in San Francisco. Lyme-literate doctors (LLMDs) were those mavericks who understood the complexity of chronic Lyme disease and had taken it upon themselves to employ long-term antibiotic protocols to treat it. These doctors belonged to the International Lyme and Associated Diseases Society (ILADS), and kept a low profile to avoid investigation by state medical boards and insurance companies who must follow the Infectious Diseases Society of America (IDSA) guidelines.

We were back in the car on yet another road trip, only this time it would be shorter—just to see Dr. Farber in San Francisco—because I was determined to get Dana back for the first week of school. She had joined the class below her for another junior year to complete the courses she missed the year before.

As we cruised north on the 405 out of Los Angeles, Dana popped a CD in the deck. A deep voice began reading the chilling book *Haunted* by Chuck Palahniuk. As the tale dove down into the darkness of sabotage, we heard Palahniuk's detailed descriptions of starvation, self-mutilation, and cannibalism.

Thirty-five minutes into it, I wailed, "I can't listen to this and drive! I feel like I'm going to vomit."

"Sometimes you need to be disturbed."

"Not now while I'm driving!"

"Oh, Momma, can't we just listen for a few more minutes? To see how it turns out?"

"I'll have to pull over and force myself to breathe—after I've thrown up!"

"All right. I'll use my ear phones." Then with a wicked smile, "I'll tell you how it turns out."

I drove in blissful silence, continuing north on Interstate 5 past the slaughterhouses, through the flat, blue-skied landscape, until I pulled into a rest stop so Dana and I could take the herbs prescribed by our Chinese herbalist. He had formulated herbs for me also, to quell the anxiety and tension I had been experiencing. We used a small spoon to scoop out the required amounts, washing them down with spring water. Back in the car Dana caught her image in the sun visor vanity mirror.

"Do you think my teeth are turning yellow from the herbs?"

I glanced in her direction. "Yes, they do look yellowish."

I checked my own in the rearview mirror. "And so do mine! Get the whitening toothpaste out of my bag!"

Dana squirted out great globs of toothpaste so we could spread it across the front of our teeth. We had to drive with our lips curled back to keep the toothpaste in place. Catching sight of each other, we literally choked back laughter as the toothpaste dribbled down our chins.

Teeth nice and white again, we sailed into San Francisco just in time for our appointment with Dr. Farber. As we walked down the grim hallway of the medical building, I smelled the mustiness of old carpet exposed to years of humid weather. The door to Dr. Farber's office had chipped paint, and just inside I spied mold in a potted plant. Somewhat reluctantly, I let the receptionist know we were there for Dana's appointment.

We sat for twenty-five minutes in the waiting room with another couple. One half of the couple, a chubby, talkative woman, sat across from us holding a stack of lab results in her hand. With some hesitation I asked her if she had Lyme disease.

"Yes." She stuck out her hand to shake mine and Dana's. "My name is Liz and this is my husband, Tom."

Dana blurted out, "Hi, I just found out I have Lyme. We've had such a hard time figuring out what's wrong with me. The doctors I've been to have all given different diagnoses. It's been driving us crazy! I'm so happy I'm here!"

"That happened to me too. What symptoms do *you* have?"

"A tightness in my chest . . . hard to breathe sometimes and an achy feeling all over my body. My head hurts and I don't think well."

With tears in her eyes, Liz replied, "I've never met anyone with my symptoms."

Dana isn't crazy after all!

When the nurse finally summoned us into a treatment room to meet Dr. Farber, Tom stood up and said with deep gratitude, "I'm so glad we met you. I hope we can stay in touch." All four of us were teary-eyed.

Dr. Farber sat at his desk in the small, unassuming office. He seemed warm and kind, like a storybook bear with brown curls and a beard. He went over Dana's labs and informed us that she had *chronic* Lyme disease because she'd had it so long, probably seven years. He explained about the use of combination antibiotics in high doses, two at a time for three months each. She would take a probiotic called Saccharomyces boulardii, a tropical strain of yeast that survived antibiotics and protected the gut. He would start her on a nine-month course to see how she did. Dana would have to take a Lyme test and complete blood count (CBC) panel every three months and come back to see him. I asked about using supplements to support her organs and immune system while she was on the antibiotics and showed him what I had in my bag, including two formulations other Lyme doctors used. He replied, "A waste of money." We left with prescriptions for the antibiotics, pain killers, and sleep medicine.

By the elevator Dana said to me, "Don't get mad, but there's mold in the waiting room at the doctor's office, and it made me feel terrible."

My blood heated. "Yes, I saw it on the windowsills and all over a plant in the bathroom."

I thought about the absurdity of the situation. How could a doctor who caters specifically to direly ill patients have an office that reeked of toxic mold? The stench made me woozy in the bathroom, where I spotted the sickly potted plant, green mold growing on the outside. How could it be that Dr. Farber hadn't made a connection between the presence of mold in his office and its negative effect on his Lyme patients, who *all* had compromised immune systems? I called his office and spoke through my teeth in my most polite voice, while inside I wanted to strike out at anyone who made Dana's hell worse.

"Do you know there is mold in your office and it is challenging for patients? My daughter got a bad headache from it today."

"We're so sorry. We're planning to remodel soon."

We arrived home from San Francisco, still reeling from the nine-month-long antibiotic protocol prescribed by Dr. Farber, and discovered George, Dana's beloved cat of fourteen years, lying on the kitchen floor almost lifeless. I immediately took him to the animal hospital, where he was put on IV fluids. Dana visited him twice that week after school, but there was little improvement. She brought George a Double Delight rose, his favorite. She placed it under his nose as we said good-bye.

I was afraid Dana's symptoms would get worse from the loss. They'd grown up together. From the beginning of her illness, George had kept her company as she lay in pain day after day on the couch. He kept a silent vigil over her, as if he knew she needed watching. The house was cold and lonely without him. In memoriam, I framed a picture of four-year-old Dana lovingly cradling baby George in her arms, and set it in the breakfast nook where he used to sleep.

Weeks went by and I found that I secretly enjoyed the house without cat hair. I resolved to be pet-free, but one day while I was out, I noticed a pet adoption across from the local post office. I was lured over by the cute puppies, thinking I could distract myself from the darkness of Dana's illness. Two tiny black kittens with green eyes immediately caught my attention. I never should have picked them up. I left but couldn't shake them from my mind. I had to tell Dana. She fell in love with them too, and they came home with us. "Betty" and "Lux" brought playfulness and delight back into our lives. They were an elixir of hope and joy.

⁕

Dana had tests every three months after her initial Lyme treatment began, and they all confirmed the presence of Borrelia burgdorferi, the Lyme spirochete. Borrelia caused an infection that disrupted many bodily processes over time and kept the immune system overtaxed. We understood it was imperative to kill the bacteria in order for all of Dana's body systems to function normally again.

After the Lyme diagnosis I became intensely involved in learning all I could about the disease. It was constantly on my mind, a nightmare that went on for days, months, and then years. I didn't know how to speak to people who asked about

Dana. In my preoccupation with the disease, I temporarily lost all sense of appropriate social behavior. I barraged anyone who would listen with technical information about the infiltrating behavior of the spirochete bacteria and the possible damage it could do to the organs, joints, nervous system, and brain. I scared myself and horrified them.

In addition to dealing with the disease itself and the ways it devastated the body, there were the incomprehensible politics of Lyme to contend with. The Center for Disease Control and Prevention (CDC) regulated Lyme treatment based on the Infectious Diseases Society of America (IDSA) guidelines, which stipulated that twenty-eight days of antibiotic treatment would kill the infection. *Period.* They claimed there was no evidence that Lyme disease was a chronic condition! However, the LDF (Lyme Disease Foundation, Inc.), cofounded in 1988 by Karen Vanderhoof-Forschner and Thomas E. Forschner, conducted scientific studies with those researchers who believed Lyme disease was serious and pervasive.

• • • • • • • • • • ⁛ • • • • • • • • •

As I slept, deep into the night, I heard Dana screaming for me. I got up and went to her room, where she sat up in bed with the covers pulled up to her eyes. Grateful to see me, she pleaded for me to turn on the light. I paused by the door, pushed the dimmer switch up, and heard her sigh.

"I'm seeing frightening creatures. They're climbing up the walls and coming towards me."

I turned up the dimmer some more, and she told me that the translucent creatures were oozing and moving by the light switch, as well as in and out of her purse. She explained that she had been practicing being creative by visualizing good things before going to sleep. When she realized her eyes were open and she could still see the creatures, she called out for me. I sat with her on her bed, as she described them and what they were doing. She was transfixed by the creatures.

What's happening? Am I witnessing a sacred initiation of some kind or a psychotic break? The creatures seemed to be like the pastel-colored "elementals" or nature spirits I'd only read about. Was Dana seeing something "real," or was this a hallucination, a manifestation of the Lyme bacteria affecting her brain and vision? It was like when she was a little girl, and we had to banish all the ghosts in her room before bed.

"I know they aren't real—I can put my hand through them."

"Tell them they can only stay if they're here to protect you."

"The scary ones have gone and now I see pink floating jellyfish all around."

I kissed her head and turned off the light. *I hate this disease. Will it take her sanity too?*

The next day Dana discovered on the internet that hallucinating was a common side effect of the sleeping pill Lunesta, which Dr. Farber had prescribed for her insomnia. She was a little disappointed thinking she would have to give up these pleasant visitations. After three days of trying other sleep medications that had no effect, we decided to try Lunesta again. Dana took half a pill, and when she couldn't sleep, she took the other half. That's when she saw the angels. I had read that in Celtic mythology the goddess "Dana" communicates with the fairies and elementals. Every night, true to her name, she visited other worlds, communicating with etheric creatures, even enlisting their guidance and protection. I imagined she was being initiated into the role of seer because I could not consider that she might be losing her mind.

In May 2009, nine months after our first visit to Dr. Farber, Dana was finally finishing up the last combination of antibiotics prescribed by him. We'd been seeing him every three months so he could check her symptoms and interpret her blood results, then prescribe the next two antibiotics. It wasn't working. Dana was not getting better; she actually seemed worse. We were losing faith in Dr. Farber's approach.

I was away at a conference for a weekend—a rare occurrence—when Dana had a scary reaction to the antibiotics. She called me, sobbing, "Mom, I'm really sick and my pee is dark." I told her to stop the antibiotics immediately, knowing this was a potential side effect of long-term antibiotic treatment, and flew home. We were once again on our own. Not only had the conventional medical approach to Lyme treatment failed to improve Dana's symptoms, but it also produced a severe and potentially life-threatening reaction. We were so naïve about what it would take to unravel this disease.

* * *

Dana was still able to hobble to high school, and began her senior year in 2009, weak but determined to graduate. During this time her relationship with her boyfriend, Aiden, was like life support. They had been friends for a long time and knew each other well. Aiden was patient with her when she was too weak or in too much pain to go out. He came over a lot after school and on the weekends. I would drive him home and occasionally pick him up at the bus stop, since neither Dana nor Aiden had their driver's licenses. One weekend Cayla came home from college to help Dana while I went away for two nights. I left everything in order: meals, rides, and medicine. They knew I'd be calling regularly to check in. Aiden would be visiting Saturday to be with Dana, which was not unusual.

When I returned Sunday afternoon, all seemed okay. Cayla hugged me good-bye on her way out to her car, carrying books and a bag of clean laundry. I made dinner for Dana while she lay resting on the couch. She seemed focused on herself, and I liked it. I felt a tiny breath of separateness between us. Dana's head hurt and her achiness was bad that night, but she slept and did not wake me. After school the next day, she called me into the living room, where she was waiting for me while I got ready to take her to her appointment with Dr. Dan, the Chinese herbalist she'd been seeing since she'd stopped Dr. Farber's protocol. When I looked at her, I saw an expression I didn't recognize, and it wasn't about physical discomfort.

"Mom, sit down here." She motioned next to her. Her face tightened. "I didn't want to have to tell you this, but I took the morning-after pill. I'm wondering if it made me sicker. I was really trying to be responsible. I thought it would be worse if I was pregnant."

Stunned—too much to take in. *She had sex!* "Oh, honey! When did you take it?"

She was worried she could be pregnant and clearly so frightened about having to tell me that I decided not to ask her what happened with the condom. My chest hurt. I felt cheated out of the talk I should have had with her. I'd postponed it because I thought she was too sick. Apparently, teenage hormones can override anything. My head was swimming. I knew she really cared for Aiden. Suddenly tears flew from Dana's eyes. She was horrified to be having this talk with me. I gave her my unconditional acceptance, and watched her slump back into the couch pillows, somewhat relieved.

"I took one of the pills at four p.m. and the other one in the middle of the night. You're supposed to take them twelve hours apart."

"Okay. Let's have Dr. Dan test you to see if the pills are interacting with his treatment."

"I don't have any more pills. There were only two pills in the package and you're supposed to take them both. They're expensive. I gave Cayla twenty-five dollars of the money you left for emergencies, and she went and got them for me."

Could the morning-after pills have made her worse? Why didn't I stay home?

"All right. We'll stop at CVS and buy a package so Dr. Dan can see if there's anything in them that might interact badly with the other meds you're taking."

"Oh no! I can't. I'll be *so* embarrassed."

"I'll go in first and explain the situation."

She threw her achy arms around me and let out a huge breath.

I ran into CVS and picked up the package, turning the box around to read the side effects list: menstrual changes, nausea, abdominal pain, tiredness, headache, dizziness, breast pain, and vomiting. *Great.*

Dr. Dan called Dana in and treated her with loving respect. He went about his usual routine of testing her body after checking the ingredients in the morning-after pill. Gently, he explained, "These pills are mostly estrogen and progestin and haven't affected you adversely."

Dana's coming-of-age experience should have been sacred, but, like most everything else at this time, it was eclipsed by her illness.

······••◦⬩◦••······

Along with physical pain, swelling, and sleep problems, hypersensitivity to sound was one of Dana's predominant symptoms. There had been a gradual descent into the rabbit hole of silence.

I came to understand the severity of this condition by reading about it on Lymeinfo.net: "Lyme disease patients can experience an extreme sensitivity to sound, also known as auditory hyperacusis. . . . In the more severe cases 'ordinary' sounds can be very debilitating. The impact can be felt throughout the body, and this condition can affect every aspect of daily living. Patients can experience heightened awareness and an inability to tolerate conversation, running water, page turning, the humming of electronic devices, other people's breathing, etc."

Every week Dana's symptoms changed, sometimes better, sometimes worse, but always persisting at a level substantiating hidden infection. I needed to accommodate the way we were actually living and make the environment of our home more comfortable for both my daughters and myself. I chose to embrace "what is" rather than continue to think that our "normal" lives were just around the corner. I came up with the genius idea of soundproof doors to separate Dana's quiet space from the rest of the house.

Two doors were installed, one between the kitchen and living room and one to my studio, which liberated Cayla and me. We could now shout or play loud music and dance, while on the other side of the doors a sacred low-sensory environment protected Dana. With Dana's healing space preserved, the kitchen came alive again and a second living room was established on the other side of the house in the studio, a place where Cayla and I could entertain friends. These doors marked a change in our lives after two years of whispering, tiptoeing, and creeping.

·······•;•·······

Dana and I were sitting together on the living room couch in the sanctuary of her quiet space. The late afternoon sun shone through a crack in the perpetually drawn curtains as silver tears ran down Dana's cheeks. I noticed every fold in the white cotton blanket between our bodies. For the past three years, she'd ached over every inch of her body, so I had barely touched her. In a blind moment I forgot everything and kissed her as a loving mother would. My lips landed on the peach-soft skin of her cheek, warm to my touch. Too warm, warm enough for a fever. She had been crying her eyes out over the life we were living. This was the first time I let go and fell into the abyss with her.

She leaned her body weakly into the big squishy couch, making an indentation that looked permanent. I wondered if she would live to sit in a new one. We were war-torn. I brushed my hand over her hair and gave her a feather-light hug, holding back. She winced. I wondered if she knew *I was with her* no matter how long it took or how hard it got.

CHAPTER EIGHT

Twins

So we grew together,
Like to a double cherry, seeming parted,
But yet an union in partition—
Two lovely berries moulded on one stem.

— William Shakespeare

D ana had been sick now for almost three years. It was December 2009, and Cayla was arriving home from her junior semester abroad in Botswana. I hadn't seen her in five months and couldn't wait! It was the holiday season, and my sister Tovya was having a big party. I wore my new, fuzzy, red chenille sweater, prepared to stop by on our way home from the airport. Cayla's flight was due to arrive at 5:00 p.m. With great anticipation I watched people sail down the escalator at LAX, scanning the crowd for Cayla's colorful exuberance. The crowd thinned out, but I didn't see her. *Had she gotten on her flight?* I started to worry as the minutes ticked by. My cell phone rang.

"Hello."

"I'm Nancy from United Airlines. Is this Anna Penenberg?"

"Yes."

"I'm calling about your daughter Cayla Penenberg. She's okay, but she has a fever and rash, and has been taken by ambulance to Wellman Medical Center. You can meet her there. Her luggage will be delivered later."

I dashed out and drove like a crazy person. The picture of the two of us swinging by the family holiday party dissolved in my mind. There was only dread.

Cayla had been isolated, and I was required to slip into a protective jumpsuit and wear a mask before I could see her. My fuzzy holiday sweater stuck out of the jumpsuit; I wasn't where I should be. I waited a heart-stopping fifteen minutes before I was finally told I could go into her room. I speed-walked down the bleached hospital corridor, my bootie-encased high heels thudding against the linoleum floors. I reached room 202 and glimpsed Cayla propped up in her bed, listing to one side, staring at the floor. She was wearing a face mask and hospital gown, her entire face and body covered in bright red spots. I made it to the other side of the doorway and collapsed on the nurse who was on her way into Cayla's room. She held me until I pulled myself together. I didn't want to scare Cayla.

"Hey, sweetie, it's so good to see you! I've missed you. Quite an outfit you came home with—spotted skin!"

Cayla mumbled to me through her face mask. "Hi, Mommy . . . I'm so hot and tired."

She seems disoriented.

Starting to sweat, I replied, "Thank God you made it home. What happened?"

"The guy next to me on my flight from DC noticed the rash on my face, so I went to the bathroom and looked in the mirror. It was bad. I got a flight attendant to help me."

"What did she do?"

"She asked over the PA system if there was a doctor on board. A nice doctor gave me Benadryl. I puked it all over myself, so the flight attendant asked me if I wanted to be taken to the hospital when we landed. I said yes."

"Good decision, honey." *Her eyes look weird—glazed and distant.*

"I don't feel good." She rolled her head to the other side of the pillow.

"I know." I couldn't stop staring at her.

"Don't worry, sweetie, the doctors are getting your blood results soon, and we'll find out what you have."

The infectious disease department at Wellman was not nearly as good as the one at Sinai General Hospital. After talking to the doctor on call, I made the decision to take Cayla to Sinai General. I penned my signature to a legal document stating that I was taking responsibility for removing Cayla from the hospital.

I asked the nurse to walk Cayla to the back door while I ran out to get the car. I pulled around to find Cayla standing outside in her skimpy hospital gown, clutching her lab results. The night air was cool so I wrapped her in my long black coat. She shivered.

"Where are your clothes?"

"They're covered in vomit."

It was twenty minutes to Sinai General, and I felt the weight of my decision now that it was just the two of us.

By the time we reached Sinai, Cayla had a 105-degree fever. She was immediately given a bed in Emergency, where we waited anxiously for news from the doctor on call. Her dad arrived and was there for the diagnosis when Dr. Amara came in twenty minutes later.

"I have reviewed Cayla's blood work, and she has rickettsia, also known as Mediterranean spotted fever."

What were the chances that both my daughters would be afflicted by tick-borne diseases? *What kind of Jobian experience am I having?*

Cayla was transferred to her own room on the sixth floor.

"Mom, the light is bothering me."

"Okay, I'll turn it down. You'll be here for a few days so they can give you IV antibiotics to get the infection under control."

Cayla's eyes were the color of red silk, shiny and bright. *Will her vision be impaired?*

When I got home that night, I researched rickettsia on the internet and read that there was indeed a possibility that her eyes could be permanently damaged. I was numb.

For four days I awoke to Dana's pressing needs, then left at 11:30 a.m., stopping at the deli for chicken soup and other treats to take to Cayla in the hospital, where she found the food lifeless and inedible.

"Mom, you're forty-five minutes late! I'm hungry. I'm not talking to you!" And she didn't for at least an hour. I couldn't be in two places at once, and I worried about the one I wasn't looking after. I moved between the tandem illnesses, trying to be there for both, never long enough for either, stretching and breaking my heart.

Cayla was also in the midst of culture shock, having just returned to the US after spending five months in Botswana, where she was learning to speak Setswana and dancing in the local traditional dance company, Mogwana. She was between cultures, living in limbo in the hospital, where no one had ever heard of Botswana.

On the fifth day, Cayla insisted on being sprung from the hospital. She was better, and the spots were diminishing, but her sensitivity to light seemed worse. Nonetheless, Dr. Amara let her go. It was her twenty-first birthday. She had such acute visual sensitivity that I had to drive her home with blackout fabric draped over her head. At home she retired to her room, drew the shades, and decided to "cancel" her birthday until she was well enough to enjoy it.

During the next few weeks, Cayla and Dana were in a parallel experience, recovering from infections that required medicine and rest. One late night I sat next to Cayla on her purple bed with big pillows. "How are you doing, hon?"

"I'm thinking about how scared I've been these last three years about Dana. She hasn't been the same since the illness. I don't understand what is happening to her. Now I'm double scared about myself."

"You will get well and recover completely in another week or two."

"I know. I feel a little better every day, but Dana doesn't. I'm having a taste of her life, and it makes me so sad. I'm angry too!"

"The best thing you could do is be kind to her as we figure out how to help her recover from this chronic illness."

"I love her and miss her being able to do things with me."

Some days later Dana and I were lounging on the couch in the living room in our pajamas while Cayla, perched in a stuffed armchair across from us, captivated us with her experiences in Botswana. She leapt off the armchair and declared, "Hey, Dana, I learned a traditional rain dance from Mogwana. We need rain. I'm going to dance for it. Watch me! And when you are better, you can dance with me!"

There she was in front of us, all five feet seven of her in orange flannel pajamas, strapping on the traditional ankle rattles made of dried seeds. Her dark hair was curled on top of her head, and her muscular arms showed through her shirtsleeves. She absolutely glowed.

"The word for rain in Setswana is *pula*. It also means blessing. When we performed this dance in Botswana, it actually rained!"

Cayla began to hum and stomp her feet, shaking the rattles. She was spinning, stomping, and crouching down in motions that made the earth want moisture. I went with her to this sacred space, where the dance was ageless—I was too. I glanced over at Dana, whose eyes were wide open, both of us enthralled by Cayla's big, bold soul. She ended with her arms up, the seeds trickling down her ankles, and bounded over to hug Dana. I expected rain.

• • • • • • • • •⸙• • • • • • • • •

To celebrate Cayla's recovery from rickettsia, we decided to go out to a movie together before she returned to college for the second semester of her junior year. She threw on a hot pink sweatshirt over a green-striped sundress, slid on dangling, diamond-shaped, purple earrings, and declared, "I'm ready for a night on the town!"

We arrived at the theater too late to get into the movie. Cayla tapped my shoulder. "The ArcLight is so stupid. It's the only theater that closes its doors when the movie starts!"

I glanced at the other movie choices. "How about seeing *Gulliver's Travels*?"

"No way, Momz! Hey! I know what we can do! There's an Indian restaurant near here, and I loooove Indian food."

"Dinner sounds good." And it did. I was ravenous!

When we entered the restaurant, the smell of curry and the plush red velvet booths made me feel cozy and even hungrier. Cayla and I were seated with dinner menus.

"Look at this menu, Mom. They have such delicious dishes here. I want some garlic naan. . . . Oh my God, they have goat!"

"Goat?"

"Yes! It says here, 'Mutton Masala.' I can't believe it! I'm so excited to have the food I ate in Botswana."

A striking, young Indian man with a beautiful smile came over to the table to take our order. Cayla asked him about the goat and he assured her it was very good.

"I'll have the Mutton Masala, please."

Cayla found it chewy, until she ate a piece that brought the taste and texture of Botswana back into her body. She sat on the red cushions chewing quietly with a far-off look in her eyes.

It was hard to believe I'd had two girls at home in pajamas with the lights turned down, recovering from tick-borne infections. The girls had twin experiences for a time, and I was oddly grateful for this twist of fate that brought the girls back together.

PART THREE

CHAPTER NINE

Message from a Tree

So Moses thought, "I will go over and see this strange sight—why the bush does not burn up."

—Holy Bible

"Dana, we have to leave *now* to get to Dr. Trudeau's! I know you don't want to go, but you promised your dad." It was the beginning of 2010, the fourth year of her illness. She was running late as usual, moving slowly. It always took her a long time to get ready. I was standing in the hallway outside her bedroom, ready to go. I heard her shuffling, so I yelled through the door, "Please hurry up!" The scent of lavender wafted into the hallway; she was almost ready.

Dana's father had decided to send her to Dr. Trudeau, a behavioral psychologist, because he had become increasingly frustrated with the unsuccessful medical treatments we'd tried. He still believed in the possibility that her illness could be psychosomatic in origin.

Two weeks earlier I had taken Dana to see Dr. Trudeau for the first time. We met the placating older man in his drab office waiting room. He wore a dark toupee on top of his wrinkled-prune face. I thought he was much too old to sympathize with a teenager. On our way home from this first session, Dana was hysterical.

"Mom, he wants me to take antidepressants! He talked down to me and treated me like I was just some moody kid! He made me feel worse. I don't want to go back to him!"

I answered in an even tone, "That's disappointing," but I was thinking I'd like to pick up the wrinkled little bastard and smash his face on the floor.

"Yeah. He told me I needed to learn how to relax, and I told him I meditate every day."

"Good."

"He told me to let him know if I want to come back. I don't."

"Okay. But you'll have to talk to your father and tell him how it went."

Dana called her father when we got home. "Dad, I really don't think Dr. Trudeau can help me. I don't want to go anymore. He even wants me to take antidepressants!"

A pause. Dana paced the hall. "I *have* given it a chance. I went to see him."

She walked into the kitchen, where I was making dinner, and gave me the *what the fuck* look while she listened to her father's lecture.

She nodded. "All right, I'll go one more time. . . . I know you're paying for it. . . . Thank you, Dad."

Clenching my keys, I walked away from Dana's door, pulled my sunglasses out of my purse, and headed toward the kitchen. I heard light footsteps behind me. Dana walked past me wearing her pink floral dress, tights, and black lace-up ankle boots. She declared, "I'm ready."

I bagged a few apples and grabbed two water bottles. "Sweetie, even though it's rush hour, I think we can still make it on time."

She sighed.

I drove straight up Jellico, took a left on Prairie, another left on White Oak, and turned onto Nordhoff Boulevard, just five minutes from the on-ramp to the 405 freeway. "Dana, if you get hungry, I brought an apple and some—"

Crash!

"Mom!"

Is the sky falling? Glass shattered around me. I was still driving. *Driving through what?* Something went by the front windshield. It was green. Pine needles. A tree branch. Lots of them. *Are we driving through a tree? What hit us?* I smelled Christmas. I saw a red sports car pass me on the opposite side of the road. The driver had his head out the window with his mouth hanging open.

This is bad. How are we going to get to Dr. Trudeau's? I have to get the windshield fixed. I was still driving. I made a left turn onto Louise Road and parked across from the house where Dana's high school English teacher lived. A beautiful country home, light blue with white trim and roses blooming.

I looked at Dana, pale and trembling, still buckled securely into her seat belt. Millions of tiny shards of glass lay everywhere inside the car, but we were not bleeding. We were untouched.

"I hope this isn't happening because you don't want to go to Dr. Trudeau's." Dana arched one eyebrow at me.

Questions flooded my mind. *Are we at war and I just can't see the enemy? Were we hit from above? Are we going to die?* All my efforts to save Dana would be lost.

A white Lexus stopped and two women got out. They came to my door and asked if we were all right. One asked, "How did that tree hit you?"

The other one shouted, "We saw it lying across three lanes."

"It's so wide, you must have driven through it after it fell on top of your car."

"A huge pine tree."

"The police are closing the boulevard."

How much time has passed? I looked at the clock in the dashboard, still intact: 5:10 p.m. Just five minutes since we left the house. My hands were shaking. I grabbed my phone and punched in Dr. Trudeau's number.

"This is Anna Penenberg. We're not able to come today. A tree fell on our car."

I punched in my insurance company's number—like I was supposed to after an accident. My agent Mischa told me to have my car towed.

A warm bear of a policeman opened my car door. He offered his hand. I was still shaking. I took his hand, climbed out, and clung on to him for a moment. He held me until I stopped shaking. The two women helped Dana get out of the car through the back door, because the front passenger door was jammed. I looked at my contorted car, pine needles and branches fused with crushed metal—a crazy Christmas wreath.

As Dana and I stood on the curb, neighbors gathered around us. There was a woman with red hair, who saw the tree fall on our car as she looked out her kitchen window while washing dishes. A pretty woman with a baby, who owned the house where the pine tree uprooted, tiptoed over. A tall man, who happened to be walking by when the tree fell, appeared. Then a chatty reporter from the Cal State Northridge newspaper stopped to interview us. I felt like a celebrity. This was newsworthy for Northridge.

A tree had come down on our moving car. A pine tree, breaking glass, smashing and bending metal. My Lexus, the one I finally owned outright. I walked to the corner with the neighbors and saw the substantial tree for myself, lying across three lanes of Nordhoff Boulevard. A wave of nausea coursed through me.

The policeman caught my attention and cautioned me not to speak to the young woman holding the baby. He lowered his voice and said, "This is now a legal issue with the city. She hired her gardener to trim her trees, not a bonded tree trimmer. She's liable for the tree that uprooted as you drove by. The idiot sawed off all the lower branches on *one* side of the tree."

The police tow truck arrived, and the driver hooked up my car.

"Wow! I've never seen a tree fall on a car," exclaimed the tow truck driver. "It's a once-in-a-lifetime experience."

"I hope so."

As we drove toward the body shop, I couldn't help but watch the large trees lining the street to make sure they were not moving off their roots. My stomach roiled. We were headed for Moses Auto Body.

Moses himself inspected my car and told me, "I can repair her, but your insurance company will probably deem her unsalvageable."

In the Bible, when Moses came upon the burning bush, he was astounded that the bush had not been consumed by the flame, just as we were astounded that we had not been crushed by the pine tree. God informed Moses that he was to lead the

Israelites out of Egypt, out of slavery to the Promised Land. *Is this where Dana and I are going? Are we leaving our fear, the illness, and the doctors' futile attempts behind? Is this our sign from God? We are listening now, on all levels.*

CHAPTER TEN

Weird Is Good!

Success is not final, failure is not fatal: it is
the courage to continue that counts.

—Winston Churchill

Dana was still experiencing hallucinations at night, a side effect of her current sleep medication, temazepam (a benzodiazepine), but when she stopped taking it, she experienced severe withdrawal symptoms and was unable to stay in school. After I started doing some research online, I discovered that it is considered harder to get off of than heroin. An internist I consulted explained that thirty milligrams is a high dose, and that the only safe way for Dana to stop using it would be for her to be weaned off it slowly over a period of five months. After some more research, we discovered there was a way to safely withdraw in only two weeks using an IV amino acid treatment. That's when my ex-husband's wife, Sheila, told us about Dr. Koozik.

"He works miracles. He can get Dana well and off her sleep medicine!"

Carting the thick file folder containing three years of lab results, I forcefully pulled open Dr. Koozik's heavy office door and marched inside with Dana in tow. We were greeted by Dana's dad, Sheila, and a short, bald man in scrubs sporting a big crooked smile—Dr. Koozik. He escorted us into a small, bland treatment room with a chiropractic table, several chairs, and IV supplies. His attention focused like a laser beam on Dana.

For the umpteenth time, she explained, "I've been sick for over three years. I feel pain all over. I have inflammation, headaches, nausea, depression, and anxiety, and I have difficulty sleeping. In the last few months, I've been hallucinating from the sleep meds I'm taking."

Dr. Koozik briefly sifted through the mountain of lab results, looked cheerfully at Dana, and confidently declared, "I'll get you feeling better soon. The doctors who treated you didn't know what they were doing. People come to me when all else fails, and I get them well."

We are in good hands! He has saved others from disease and death. He's a miracle worker, and Dana will soon be as good as new. I felt like I just performed a perfect flip off the high dive.

Dr. Koozik said, "I'm going to give Dana IV amino acids to get her off the sleep medicine." Then he stated with authority, "She doesn't have Lyme."

I couldn't believe what he was saying. I *wanted* to believe what he was saying! In that moment I decided to let go of all panic about bacteria stealthily killing my daughter. I let go of the monster Lyme disease and gratefully surrendered to Dr. Koozik's diagnosis. He noted that the most recent Lyme panel read "negative." I wanted so badly to trust Dr. Koozik that I disregarded the fact that blood test results for Lyme patients who have been on antibiotics will often come back with a false negative. Dr. Koozik assured me that he knew all about Lyme infections. It was *so* good to let go.

As soon as my ex-husband and his wife left the office, Dr. Koozik's professional manner dissolved. He looked at Dana. "Now that your dad is gone, we can party! I'm going to give you IV vitamin C to chelate your toxins and acupuncture to start building up your system. It's fucking stupid what the doctors have been doing with you for the last three years."

Dana and I looked at each other and smiled. I relaxed for the first time in three years and let *him* call the shots. Two days later we came back for more IV treatments. I sat for two hours watching fluids pour through a clear plastic tube into Dana's arm. She was Dr. Koozik's prize patient. He was out to impress Dana's father by curing her illness.

Dana improved and got stronger. She began going for short walks every day. I hoped she might actually be able to get off the couch, where she had been resting day and night, and return to her classes again. Treatments continued three times a week.

Dr. Koozik explained to us one day that he also practiced "energy medicine," a fact he had not shared with my ex and his wife. As he waved his hands over Dana's body, she said, "This feels weird. I feel a cold sensation draining from my head."

"Weird is good!" Koozik beamed. We soon learned that this was his mantra.

"Dr. Koozik, what did you clear?"

"Something from a past life."

"Oh, what was it?"

"Well, shit. It was a life where you fell in love with a boy from another village. The families didn't get along and wouldn't allow you to be together. You poisoned the water source to his village and killed them all."

Dr. Koozik was undoubtedly flamboyant and dramatic, but I wondered at this moment whether he might actually be crazy. I peeked over at Dana and she grinned. She and I both wanted these treatments to work.

During the third week of her treatments, Dr. Koozik said, "Dana, I'm going to treat you with ozone therapy at my clinic in Mexico. It's currently illegal to administer ozone in California, but I promise you that it's completely safe and will eradicate the infection from your body." He then looked at me and winked. "We won't tell Dana's dad."

Dana's eyes narrowed as she looked up at Koozik. "What is ozone therapy and how will it affect my body?"

"It's a process in which blood is cycled out of one arm, filtered, oxygenated with ozone, and run back into the body through the other arm. This goes on for about an hour and is a very thorough way to kill infectious disease and remove accumulated toxins. You should feel much better after a few treatments."

Dr. Koozik then looked at me and said, "Dana will have to go down to Mexico for these treatments, possibly once or twice a week for about fifteen visits."

It was getting weirder and weirder. Was weird good? Could it be that this grandiose little man with the charisma of a drug lord would be the one to set Dana free?

<hr/>

Dana's first ozone treatment was scheduled on the first day of Passover. It was significant to me that the celebration of the liberation of the Jews three thousand years ago and our journey toward freedom from the enslaving illness arrived simultaneously. My family had eaten the ritual Passover meal and told the story of the exodus from Egypt since I was a child. I told my family we would not be there for the Seder dinner. I hoped our liberation would take place over the border in Mexico and be the beginning of the last phase of my daughter's recovery.

We drove two hundred miles in my new Honda CRV to cross the border into Tijuana, where a plethora of medical clinics served American patients seeking treatments that were illegal in the US. We parked in San Diego and walked through the swinging metal door into Mexico. Rising up to meet us as we entered Tijuana were the savory, sweet aromas of menudo, tortillas, and churros, blended with the acrid stench of sewage. We hired a taxi and rode the five minutes to the clinic without any difficulty.

The front door to the clinic opened into a bright, fluorescent-lit room featuring four different shades of blue paint. On the table next to the waiting room chairs was a stack of brochures for Postday, a Mexican morning-after pill. *Why are women's fertility issues being addressed in this office?* A female patient with enormous breasts walked out of the doctor's office. Her saccharine perfume wafted by as she clicked along in her stiletto-heeled boots. Her see-through sweater showed off her white, industrial-strength bra. *Where are we?*

Fifteen minutes later we received kisses from plump Nurse Lucinda, who was overflowing with love and generosity of spirit. Dana walked into the treatment room and made herself comfortable in the recliner. Lucinda skillfully inserted a catheter into each of Dana's arms, then turned on the square, metal ozone machine, which droned loudly. After she attached clear plastic tubes from Dana's catheters to the ozone machine, she patted the "out" tube to help Dana's clotted blood course through. Dana's blood flowed out of one tube, traveled through the machine where it was cleaned and oxygenated, and then returned in the other tube.

I made my way to the waiting room to relax for a while. Periodically I peeked in, and as I watched Dana's blood circulate through the machine, bubbles of sweat formed on my face and under my arms. She looked so small and frail in the big padded chair. Heartache coursed through me.

By our fourth trip, Lucinda could not get a needle into Dana's arm veins.

"Dana, I'm going to use the top of your hands for a vein. It is more sensitive here."

Lucinda cut off the red Buddhist prayer string tied onto Dana's wrist. It was meant to fall off on its own when the prayer was no longer needed. When we left the clinic, I worried about the ozone vapors she had inhaled from a flaw in the machine. She was coughing and had chest pain, and wrinkles appeared around her eyes as she labored to breathe. *Will this get worse? Will I need to rush her to a doctor as soon as we get back over the border?*

It took Dana several days to recover from the inhalation of ozone, so I decided she would wear an oxygen mask during her sessions from then on. In spite of this glitch, she felt better for the first time a few days following the treatment, which convinced us that more treatments could make her feel even better.

Not long after Dana's seventh trip to the clinic in Mexico, she became weak all over. She had terrible pain coming from what she thought was her liver, and wasn't sleeping. The doctor we were putting all our faith in was out of the country, out of cell range, and out of touch. We had no way of finding out whether we should go ahead with the next ozone therapy appointment. Dr. Koozik had promised us Dana would heal with these treatments in Mexico.

I realized Dr. Koozik didn't know what he was dealing with. I still wanted to believe Dr. Koozik's claim that Dana didn't have Lyme disease, but deep inside I suspected she was still riddled with Lyme bacteria. I couldn't imagine another day with the devastating possibility that we were not even close to winning the war we'd been waging. *Is the extreme swelling going to lead to kidney failure? And why is she so swollen? Has the ozone damaged her?* I was overwhelmed by the enormous responsibility on my shoulders. I postponed the next ozone therapy appointment and took Dana to our internal medicine doctor for liver and kidney function tests.

Two days later, after the internist reviewed her results, he called to say that everything was within normal range. We braved the trip to Mexico, hoping the next ozone treatment would relieve Dana of the inflammation that plagued her. She had gained eight pounds in one month.

After her treatment, we rode back to the border with an American woman, also one of Dr. Koozik's patients. As I chatted with her, I became increasingly aware of her stretched face, plump immovable lips, and ample bosom jutting out into the steering wheel. She made small talk about our doctor, whose clinic, it turned out, is in fact renowned for its "antiaging" treatments. *Oh my God, I'm taking my daughter to a Mexican cosmetic clinic for a serious illness!*

Dana was getting worse and an old rash reappeared, along with even more swelling. Dr. Koozik avoided my questions about Lyme bacteria and had no understanding of the characteristic rash on her leg. He was out of the country, yet again, and we were scheduled for another ozone therapy treatment. I sent him an email with carefully selected notes from Lyme specialist Dr. Burrascano on the behavior of Lyme bacteria:

> Undertreated infections will inevitably resurface, usually as chronic Lyme, with its tremendous problems of morbidity and difficulty with diagnosis and

treatment. . . . Other key symptoms may include gastritis . . . and red rashes. These rashes may have the appearance of red streaks like stretch marks. . . . Borrelia burgdorferi (Lyme) can change from the spiral form ("spirochete") into a cyst form. This cyst seems to be able to remain dormant (as long as ten months), but when placed into an environment more favorable to its growth, Bb can revert into the spirochete form. (Advanced Topics in Lyme Disease: Diagnostic Hints and Treatment Guidelines for Lyme and Other Tick Borne Illnesses, by Joseph J. Burrascano Jr., MD)

Although I hoped the information about inactive states of Lyme would make Dr. Koozik look at Dana's case from a new perspective, Dana begged me not to question him. She couldn't tolerate any doubt on my part. She desperately needed to believe he was making her well.

We drove to the Mexico clinic for the twelfth time in less than a year. Dana didn't feel good and took it out on me with deadly silences and grumbling about anything I did that unintentionally caused her more discomfort.

"What did you put on your hair? It's giving me a headache!"

"Just shampoo."

"Ugh . . . it's awful." She turned up the volume on the stereo. Angry, punk rock screamed from the speakers.

"Dana, can you please put on something more mellow?"

"This *is* mellow!"

I blocked it out and forced myself to drive the speed limit for the next four hours.

Just after we arrived at the Mexico clinic, Dr. Koozik unexpectedly walked through the door and stepped behind the reception desk without acknowledging us. He kept answering cell phone calls that rang with the macho *Rocky* theme song. I seethed quietly in my seat, feeling invisible. Dr. Koozik peeked into the treatment room to tell Dana she looked good, then nodded to me as he passed back out through the lobby. He didn't talk to me and never addressed any of my concerns about Lyme. *Has he even read my email?*

Dana slumped in the recliner for an hour as her dark, thick blood flowed out and back in, refreshed and oxygenated. Dr. Manuel (Dr. Koozik's Mexican colleague) took patient calls and talked loudly into his phone in Spanish, his voice echoing through the carpetless rooms. The young receptionist was bored and used his lunch chopsticks to beat out complicated drum rhythms that rang through the clinic, making it impossible for me to relax.

Dana had chosen to forgo the oxygen mask, a "fuck you" to me. As a result, the window in the treatment room was wide open. When I checked on her, flies were dancing in the air above her head. She hated me to hover. I hated her to be sick and I hated taking her to Mexico. We made the long trip home in silence.

Dana and I were in deep conflict over Dr. Koozik. She felt secure with him and trusted his every word. Although Dana had made significant improvement during the first four months, I thought his treatments were ultimately proving to be ineffective. He had no real knowledge of Lyme disease and was treating her like she had benign bacteria that could be easily eradicated. I believed that the Lyme disease resided deep in Dana's system and that it would take skill and experience to combat the chronic infestation. She was caught in the middle; she liked the attention she got from Dr. Koozik. He made grand promises to get her well, and repeatedly told her that she is "better than she thinks," even while her symptoms were getting worse.

At home in Northridge where the kitchen smelled like steamed greens and the afternoon light gave it a warm, patchy glow, Dana stood at the chopping block island leaning over her meal.

"What am I going to do?"

"About what?"

"About my treatment. I know you don't want to take me to Mexico anymore." Tears roll down her swollen face, the excessive puffiness alerting me to the emotional stress she was under.

I looked at her through loving eyes and said, "I just don't feel good about it. I don't know if the treatment is helping. I need more information, more answers to my questions."

"Well, you need to call Dr. Koozik and ask him yourself—now!"

So I made the call. Koozik explained, "The ozone is pushing the infection out of the deep tissues. She needs more IV amino acids and I haven't been giving them to her because of your financial limitations and it's slowing down her recovery." Blah, blah, blah, about how he wasn't making any money treating Dana, and how she needed to continue the ozone treatments to get well. I walked back into the fading light of the kitchen and saw Dana sitting next to Betty, petting her gently.

She caught the irritation in my face and whimpered, "What are we going to do?"

I caved. I ran to hold her, both of us sobbing, caught in a complex tangle of love, money, emotions, and disease. I could have burned the city down with my thoughts. I despised this illness that threatened to destroy what I loved most in this life, my child. I hated being a fugitive from my own life. I hated what it had done to my daughter's body. I hated being alone in this. I wanted to stop this hard life, this horror, this prison, this deprivation.

I missed things I would never have dreamed mattered so much, like laughing with friends in my own home, like having a whole hour without worrying. Nothing soothed me anymore, not my baths, romance novels, music, or deeply cherished garden.

Dana and I made a compromise. I would no longer take her to Mexico, and since she was not ready to quit seeing Dr. Koozik, she would go to her appointments in his LA office by herself. I did not want to be there anymore, and Dr. Koozik didn't want me in the treatment room. I asked too many questions he wouldn't or couldn't answer. I was willing to make this compromise because I believed the IV vitamin treatments he was giving her not only couldn't do her any harm but were supportive to her healing.

At this point Dana began to decline rapidly. She had stomachaches, panic attacks, and more difficulty than ever sleeping. Not only would Dr. Koozik refuse to answer her texts, he was unkind to her during her appointments. The crazy doctor we'd had so much fun with in the earlier phase of Dana's treatments had become the devil. What had been quirky and outlandish before was no longer amusing.

I had Dana's blood and urine tested again. The urine showed a high white cell count, indicating active infection. I delivered the test results to Dr. Koozik, who ignored me but was smart enough to know what I understood from the results. He didn't say anything to me, but Dana informed me later that he had given her an IV antibiotic for Lyme, because he said the Lyme infection had come back a little. He told her she would need to have an IV antibiotic administered three times a week for three weeks.

Bullshit! Lyme does not come back "a little"! She's had it all along, and Dr. Koozik never understood the nature of the disease, or how to treat it.

Dana's decline continued. I found out that the antibiotic Dr. Koozik had been administering was no longer used by Lyme doctors! I watched Dana's life force being sucked out of her. I felt like destroying Koozik's office and smashing in his smug face, but I was afraid to interfere because I knew Dana would be angry with me. Fortunately, she finally saw Dr. Koozik for who he was, a dangerous man full of his own "genius." He was *always* right. People who questioned his methods were "too whiny." She saw how he had preyed on her vulnerability. He claimed to be the one master who could rout out any toxin or cure any illness, but when all he could tell her time after time was "you're detoxing," she began to understand that he didn't know what was wrong with her or how to help her. Dana had been sucked into this relationship, and his manipulations had eaten away at her sense of self.

With determined tears streaming down her face, she declared, "I hate Dr. Koozik! *I'm* going to be in charge from now on!"

Weird was not good. Weird was just weird.

CHAPTER ELEVEN

Moxie

Once you make a decision, the universe
conspires to make it happen.

— Ralph Waldo Emerson

Dana was a buoyant baby, and as a toddler she had to have everything her way and would have loud tantrums when it wasn't possible. I held her yelling and kicking one day at the bakery counter while I picked up a pie for dessert. She scared the line of people waiting to buy bread and pastries, but I held her tight, trying to teach her that she could not always override me. We made it out with the pie intact. Down the road she slipped out of the belts of her child seat and stood on the back bench. I adored her even as I screamed at her to sit down. So much determination poured out of her.

She was a curious second grader, sturdy and tall for her age with long, straight dark hair and a face-covering smile. Her class was studying rain forests and had decorated the ceiling of their classroom with colorful crepe paper trees and raindrops. Dana would not stop talking about rain forests. She begged me, "Mommy, can we *please* go visit the rain forest?"

Her pleading made me think seriously about taking a family vacation that we would remember the rest of our lives. Dana was eight and Cayla ten. Maybe this was a good time to go see the world together. As it happened, my sister Tovya owned an adventure travel business. She put me in touch with her colleague, who led trips into the Manu Biosphere Reserve in the Amazon. A *real* rain forest! We talked our friends Gertie and Mike into coming with us. Cayla and Dana were friends with their kids, Melanie and Mitch. With four adults and four kids, we officially qualified as a group and would be able to hire our own personal guides to lead us into the Amazon and around Cusco and Machu Picchu. We were all excited.

Several months later, after acquiring the right clothing and equipment for the hot climate, pills to prevent malaria, herbal sprays for mosquitoes, passports, and visas, we boarded a direct flight to Lima, Peru. Upon arrival we were met by our guide, Jesus, and taken to our hotel. He was a solid man with a warm smile and a sweet connection with our kids. He briefed us about everything we were going to see and do, and warned us about altitude sickness. The next morning we flew to Cusco, the historic capital of the Inca Empire situated at eleven thousand feet. After we drove to the hotel on a narrow cobblestone street, Jesus gave us cocoa leaf tea to take the edge off the light-headedness we were all experiencing. There in the invigorating city of Cusco, alive at night with music and brightly colored clothing, we began our adventures.

Led by our Quechuan shaman, Apo, we toured Machu Picchu, drove through the Urubamba Valley, and climbed through Ollantaytambo, the archaeological site of an Incan

Emperor's royal estate. Then, with our minds and hearts expanded, we flew in a chartered ten-seater plane with our belongings, our curiosity, and enough food and drinking water for nine days in the Amazon jungle. We were on our way to see Dana's rain forest! The plane landed in a field where a native man in a white loincloth came running to meet us. From then on we traveled by canoe.

Down the river and deep into the forest, we stopped to visit a tribe. This was the last sign of civilization we would see for days. There was a tiny store and large grassy field in the middle of the village. Our kids played on soccer teams at home and jumped at the invitation to play with the native children. Among them was a skilled soccer player named "Hitler." We were appalled by the idea that this was considered a mighty name to bestow on an Amazonian tribal son in the 1990s. Our kids held their own, even in the humid heat, but the shoeless team from the village ultimately took the lead. We celebrated outside the tiny store by buying cold drinks for everyone.

Back in our sturdy canoe, motoring through the Madre de Dios River, we passed white caimans (alligators) sleeping on the banks, a family of otters, turtles, and many kinds of birds, including herons, egrets, Orinoco geese, terns, and skimmers. The banks were dense with lush foliage and towering trees rising above their visible roots. Piranhas were plentiful in this river as well as sunken tree trunks. It was the responsibility of our native boat guide to carefully navigate around the hidden dangers. Our lives were in his hands.

On a predawn river trip out to a boathouse on the water, we asked our overexcited children to observe silence so we could watch the scarlet macaws feed at a spot on the shoreline where the cliffs were made of salty clay. We didn't want our voices to scare them away. Once at the boathouse we hunkered down to wait, munching on snacks, while the kids quietly entertained themselves by drawing. Dana was busy working, crouched on the floating wooden floor, her favorite colored pencils rolling to the side of her paper. She drew with a fierce concentration that kept her engaged in the fine details of her work. At dawn we were blessed with a display of scarlet macaws. Looking out the openings in the boathouse, we were enchanted by the fluttering of their brightly colored wings. They would perch and lick the salt off the cliff edge, one of the few places in the world where they congregate like this. Our children were spellbound.

We stayed at a jungle lodge deep in Manu, our farthest destination and definitely the nicest accommodations, after having spent the majority of our trip in *M*A*S*H*-like tent camps. Our rooms rested on pilings above the jungle floor, and our beds were surrounded by mosquito netting. On the first day, we encountered a monkey who came right up to us and even climbed on Mitch's shoulders. Prior to this encounter we'd spent many long days walking on trails searching for wildlife and looking through binoculars up into tall trees for monkeys. Cameras snapped away as Dana jumped up and down, enjoying our miracle. At dinner that night it became apparent that our monkey, Arturo, was the trained personal pet of the lodge owner. Nevertheless, it was a real treat.

We prepared for our biggest expedition: an overnight at the den of the tapir—large, gentle prehistoric creatures with big snouts. We couldn't wait. With four excited children, packs full of dinner, snacks, flashlights, and extra clothes, we padded down the two-mile path in silence. We had been given instructions to be as quiet as possible because sounds in the jungle could travel for up to a mile. The goal was to sneak into the special tent rooms built on wooden platforms specially designed for watching the nocturnal tapirs at their watering hole. During the hike, Mitch, the youngest, asked many questions in his piercing whisper as the other children's giggles echoed through the forest. It seemed silence caused laughter, and whispering made noise. We hushed the children, feeding them snacks and hoping we had been quiet enough.

When the silence lasted only a short while, Dana whispered in my ear, "Mom, make them stop! The tapirs will hear us and I want to see them!" She tapped Mitch's shoulder and swept her hand across her lips.

Dana continued to march along in silence, staying true to our mission—her long hair swinging in a ponytail, her blue backpack hanging from her small shoulders, and her photographic eyes focusing on the trail. We arrived at the site, climbed into our places, and lay down to wait. Dana stayed awake the longest of all the children, until finally her eyelids gave up the fight. We didn't see the brown, fuzzy tapir that night, but the kids slept soundly in the jungle air even with the constant soundtrack of squawking birds. I let go of my disappointment because the entire trip had been extraordinary. Dana's intense desire had translated into a thrilling adventure.

CHAPTER TWELVE

Pomp and Extraordinary Circumstance

In art and dream may you proceed with abandon.
In life may you proceed with balance and stealth.

— Patti Smith

Dana's Waldorf school supported the development of the whole person. Its philosophy was based on Rudolf Steiner's art of learning experientially through the heart, head, and hands. Every year, several weeks before graduation, the senior class and their parents participated in a final council meeting guided by a faculty member. Council, a form of communication used in grades six through twelve, taught the students honest self-expression in a safe environment. One person spoke at a time, "briefly and from the heart." Dana and I had been looking forward to this school ritual, but she was too sick to attend the night of the meeting, so I agreed to go without her.

Debra, the facilitator for the evening, asked us all to sit down—parents in the outer circle and senior students in the inner circle facing their parents. Debra placed a chair in front of me, even though Dana would not be sitting in it that evening.

Debra began the ritual by asking the parent sitting next to me to start: "Ronald, please speak to your son about what you know of him and what you wish for him as he moves on from high school."

Suddenly I was next. All I could manage was "I'll pass."

Debra leaned in. "Why don't you speak to Dana as if she were here before you?"

My face flushed; everyone was now looking at me. I felt I would break apart. I wanted to refuse, to wait until the others talked with their children, but the parents motioned for me to speak. I was unprepared; I didn't know what would come out. I looked at the empty chair and visualized Dana seated before me. She was beautiful and slender, her hair was down, hanging softly around her face, and she was feeling her best.

"You are a strong person, Dana. You have faced your challenges with determination and a powerful will to always do as well as you can. You are the most courageous person I know. My wish is for you to grow into all of your potential. You *will* graduate with your class."

I then turned to everyone in the room. "Two years ago you welcomed Dana into your class when she needed more time to finish eleventh grade. Thank you for loving and accepting her just as she is. The blessing of your support has meant so much to me and Dana." I was flooded with gratitude, my red face moist with tears.

The night before graduation, the senior class presented a final play highlighting their talents through song, dance, performance, and writing. Dana was to perform and made it out of bed with sterling determination, despite having missed the critical rehearsals. She performed in a saucy dance number from the musical *Chicago*, in which she was swung upside down by her dance partner. Her shiny black hair flew and her long legs flashed as she extended them into the splits at the end of the number. I was joyously proud, happily forgetting that her strength and vigor in that moment might not last.

On graduation day Dana, dressed in a navy silk dress embellished with flowers and lace, sat with her twenty-three classmates in the middle of a semicircle. The early evening sunlight cast shadows across their faces, and the scent of jasmine permeated the entire garden. I noticed the shine on Dana's forehead moments before it was her turn to step up to the podium to deliver her graduation speech. I sat in the first row where the view was unobstructed. My sister Jain, who was there with me, took my hand and held it until the end of the ceremony.

Dana's spirit drove her up to the podium. She was a natural beauty, with her hair piled on top of her head in an elegant braided bun. No one suspected the illness underneath.

Her confident voice rang out with thoughts well beyond her years. Dana had kept her speech to herself, so I was hearing it for the first time. *Oh my God, she's such a good writer! I love her so much.* My heavy heart burst open and filled with pride as I squeezed my sister's hand.

> *I was warmly welcomed when I came to Highland Hall in fifth grade by the smaller versions of my closest friends to this day. A world of color and beauty was unveiled here, and school was a celebration of both living and learning.*

As she recalled her first experiences, a flood of relief overtook me. *She's safe in herself.*

Each class of the day was a gift, wrapped in thoughtful verses, with joy and knowledge inside. It was magnificent and I had never known anything like it. I fondly recall lying in the grass at recess, rushing down the hill when the mulberries were in season, dancing in the mud when it was rainy, silences during class to hear the seed pods pop, and water fights in the heat of spring.

Each day was an opportunity to stretch our imaginations, to push ourselves, to enjoy the differences in each other, and to build strong relationships that would have the foundation to last for the rest of our lives. In eighth grade I was given the opportunity to explore choreography, learn about the dancers that I looked up to, and choreograph and perform my own piece.

There were few dry eyes as she spoke about her "life's curriculum," inside and outside of school, surprising those who knew her, as well as those who didn't, when they realized the challenge her illness presented.

My particular path through high school was an unusual one. My education equally took place inside and outside of the classroom. The curriculum was seemingly granted by my teachers and by the universe. It was a woven journey through the teachings of academics and community alternating with the wisdom of solitude and pain.

My illness asked of me why I was living, and how much fighting living was worth. I discovered that I was living for every person who was fighting for me. After contemplating all possibilities, I made

the decision to fight for myself, and therefore also live
for myself.

Dana had made it with her soul intact and a strong will
to live. After fearing for so long that the illness would destroy
Dana's innocent joy, she'd become even more herself.

PART FOUR

CHAPTER THIRTEEN

Narrows

When we are no longer able to change a situation,
we are challenged to change ourselves.
— Viktor E. Frankl

After Dana graduated from high school, she was stable enough to be without me for a week, so I left her in the care of a close friend while I went on a group hiking trip to Zion National Park in the fall of 2010. Dana and I had driven through the park two and a half years before, but she had only seen the sights from the car windows because she'd been too sick to walk around. I wanted to go back; I wanted to hike every trail and look out from every peaked vantage point. I was craving relief from the emotional stress I lived with every day. I needed a strenuous physical challenge to deliver me back to myself.

The group would be trekking into a slot canyon in the park called the Narrows. It is a sixteen-mile stretch of the

Virgin River where the two-thousand-foot-high canyon walls get closer and closer to each other as you walk, wade, and swim into the narrowest section of the canyon. I was mesmerized by internet photos of hikers wading through the river into the steep slot canyon. The vibrant reflection of sunlit water onto carved canyon walls went straight into me, right off the screen. I had to go there.

The day I left for Utah, a storm blew in and sat over the Colorado Plateau precisely where I was headed. It was a flashing, booming thunderstorm, dumping more rain than usual. The bus ride from the Las Vegas airport felt like a feat of survival. I found myself white-knuckling as we drove through sheets of water on a winding mountain road with a sheer drop-off on one side. When the bus finally stopped for a bathroom break at a tiny gas station, I got out and ran to the bathroom as the gale force winds drove water and mud up my pants. I was thoroughly exhausted when we finally arrived safely in St. George later that night.

In the morning I met our trip leaders, Trish and Valerie, and asked, "What are our chances of going into the Narrows?"

"Well, it's presently closed to hikers due to the height of the river and possible flash floods. But anything is possible!"

We all went out hiking that first morning after being instructed on safety procedures should lightning surprise us on the trail: "Do not stand near a tree on the top of a mountain, throw your hiking poles one hundred yards away from where you're standing, and get down low."

We trudged in the pouring rain, which reddened the rock and made creeks come alive. I felt myself smiling gleefully as my body was enveloped by the cascading rainwater—a glorious natural cleanse! I looked out on the vast depth and grandeur of the stone canyons, vivid umber, ocher, and sienna streaks emerging as rain washed the glazed rock. Slogging through mud in my dripping-wet rain gear, I understood that the power of nature was far greater than we were. We got showered as we walked under a newly formed waterfall cascading off a rock ledge above us, just before we had to turn back at a stream crossing where the water was now high enough to take lives.

On our second day on the trail, my hat served as an umbrella as I hiked up to Observation Point in a downpour. Fear of lightning dictated a brief stay at the top. The sound of dripping water came and went, and patches of sunlit blue sky popped in and out as we switchbacked down the mountain. I prayed for the rain to stop and the river to calm down so we could enter the Narrows. I checked the internet: "Flash floods can occur anytime. If the river flow is over 150 cubic feet per second, no one will be allowed in. Under ideal conditions the flow is less than 70 cubic feet per second. Chest-deep holes are common, even when the river is low. Be prepared to swim." *Okay. Wow.*

We arose on the morning of our third day with good news: the trail through the river to the Narrows was open! But the water was high, flowing at 150 cubic feet per second. I figured if the National Park allowed us to go in, I was game. After a morning hike up to Angel's Landing and a picnic lunch, we arrived at the Temple of Sinawava, a magical wall of reddish stone with a waterfall cascading down through a crevice. From there we walked the mile trail toward the entry point to the river walk. On the landing overlooking the path that dropped into the river, I got my first glimpse of the swollen waters dashing over boulders.

When we got to the edge of the brown river, bubbling with white caps, a fellow hiker, Phil, offered to go first. I agreed. He's six feet two and strong. I trusted him and chose my steps by the watermarks on his knees and thighs, which on me were much higher. I thought I was prepared in my tennis shoes and neoprene socks, but a shock of cold blasted through my body as I stepped in the water. I stopped to bundle up, zipping myself into the cocoon of my fleece jacket. The strong current pulled on my legs, forcing me to use my hiking poles as extra limbs to secure my tenuous balance while I dragged each leg through the current. I felt the powerful meshing of wills, the river's and mine.

After the first two shallow crossings, several people turned back when the river deepened. We became an army of four, moving through the cloudy current, navigating unseen depths and large stones. I was relieved when the slower few quit; I resented being held back by others. Liberated to forge ahead, the four of us gained speed through the middle of the canyon as the walls moved closer and closer together. My heart pounded as I was drawn in.

Upriver I stepped onto a sandy bank and my leg disappeared to the height of my knee in quicksand formed by the new silt. Without thinking, I put my other foot down to leverage myself out, and it too was sucked out of sight into the quicksand. Phil had gone another way around the large boulder, which blocked me from view. When I shouted "Help!" his strong hands came out of nowhere and yanked me up onto the rock. I sat there, feeling the sensation of darkness drain out of me. Phil kept hold of my hand, steadying me, as a sharp rush of adrenalin caused me to shiver uncontrollably for a few minutes.

I want this so badly—to be rescued.

Before I left home, a rash had appeared on Dana's knee, indicating the probability of rampant infection. I couldn't, wouldn't, admit to myself that Dana wasn't getting better. I couldn't endure the hopelessness. I was in the river with sand and mud up to my thighs, wrestling it all out. Phil tapped me on the shoulder. I stood up tall and gathered my equilibrium. Phil offered his hand and guided me down to a solid spot of earth.

I moved ahead with the group into the narrowing canyon, witnessing the warm sunlight as it reflected off the upper walls of rust and gold stone. The group stopped at a place where our leader said we must turn back in order to make it out before dark.

No! I couldn't go back yet. "May I take a few moments alone?" I asked our leader.

"You have ten minutes before we head back. Please be careful!"

The hard-packed sandbar across from this narrow point in the river went on for some yards into the canyon, zigzagging away from my group. The wind attacked my face, the current pulled on my legs, and the rocks and boulders tipped me off balance. I began to wake up. *These are my legs, this is my life, and I am still here.*

I had an urge to run from sandbar to sandbar, faster and faster, toward what, I didn't know. Maybe to be swallowed up. Still, I trusted my instincts. I came to the end of the sandbar as it hit the sheer, solid rock wall and melted into the narrowing river. I reached out, touching the massive stone with both hands, and my whole body gave way into it. I found myself moving along the wall, splashing my way forward, hugging the cliffs. I stood on a boulder and began waving my arms in an arc above my head, scooping the air around me, inhaling and exhaling in some kind of instinctive ritual.

Soon my voice filled the canyon with tones that were neither songs nor melodies. *Where in me is this coming from?* Water rushed by, leaves murmured, the wind combed my cheeks. In the next moment, sunlight struck my chest as it slivered down between the jagged heights of stone. *It has chosen me.* Warmth filled my chest with the bright light. Silent cymbals clashed. *This* was my moment. My heart pounded and pounded and pounded. *I'm not broken.*

CHAPTER FOURTEEN

Sonic Boom

*All I ever wanted was to reach out and touch another human
being not just with my hands but with my heart.*

— Tahereh Mafi

It was April 2011, a year since Dana graduated and a week
since she stopped seeing Dr. Koozik, and we were in the car
again on yet another road trip. Four and a half hours down a
long straight road through the desert, a mindless meditation,
traveling to yet another healing treatment. This time we were
driving to Las Vegas to see a man named Ed, an engineer
who developed a sonic device we hoped would alleviate Dana's
inflammation and pain. The device was engineered so that sonic
waves traveled in and around the body, stimulating healthy
cellular function. The sound frequencies could go where oral
medications couldn't. Every cell in the body was simultaneously
stimulated, which was something pathogens couldn't tolerate.
It was brilliant!

Ed was still experimenting with the effects his sonic treatments had on Lyme patients. We were following in the footsteps of Amber, a twenty-year-old woman with Lyme we'd befriended through the online Lyme community. Ed's sonic treatments had significantly reduced Amber's Lyme disease symptoms, and she'd regained her health enough to return to her life and only needed tune-up treatments once a month. When Amber first started the treatments, she did them for one hour, twice a day, for a series of four days at a time. She kept this up for one year. I had spoken many times with her cheerful, encouraging mom, Betsy, a no-nonsense woman who boosted my spirits. The camaraderie of another mom reignited my hope for Dana's full recovery.

It was hot, dry, dusty, and windy when we arrived at Ed's office in a strip mall in Las Vegas. He was a short, balding, kind, yet inappropriately frank, streetwise ex-New Yorker. Without ceremony, he greeted us and began immediately briefing us on the treatment.

"It's very simple. For an hour you'll listen to music or rest while the sound waves fill the room." He turned to me and said, "Anna, why don't you give it a try too? It will relax you after the long drive."

Ed escorted us into the treatment room, the secret chamber. The device, a large chimney made out of speakers, sat in the center of the room with four brown leather recliners surrounding it. Dana and I each climbed into a recliner. Ed gave us noise reduction earphones to block the dull sound of the machine.

Tired from the drive, I fell asleep. Once again I dreamt that this was the cure. *Dana is dancing in a ballet recital, wearing red taffeta and white voile. Her graceful limbs glide through the air effortlessly.* At the end of the session, Ed came to get us. I was calm and felt a pleasant sensation all through my body. Dana was achy and exhausted.

When we checked in at the hotel, I was shown three worn but utilitarian suites and picked the best one. Even this nonsmoking room had to be aired out. I wiped down the counters, cabinets, side tables, desks, and chairs, as well as the entire kitchenette and bathroom with Dr. Bronner's mint-scented castile soap, and then sprayed lavender water all around the room before Dana came in. My gut clenched as I worried about all the things that might bother her. It was an impossible task to get everything just right.

After Dana settled in the bedroom where she could shut the door, I sat down in the living area to relax before dinner. I thought I'd watch a movie to distract myself. When I couldn't get the TV to turn on, I noticed the back of the remote was bare and without batteries. I wouldn't get to watch *Little House on the Prairie*, a salve for my broken dreams. Our room wasn't receiving Wi-Fi either. I marched down to the office numerous times to complain in person, and finally obtained a working remote, but no Wi-Fi.

We ate a cold dinner because the stove had a smell that made Dana scream. She was cranky, swollen, and achy, but I was still charged with hope—giddy, even. *The treatment must be flushing out the infection, which is why Dana feels so bad.* (When Lyme bacteria die, they emit neurotoxins that make one feel terrible.) Before we left Ed's treatment center, he confirmed that people generally felt worse after the first treatment or two. "Dana will turn a corner." This phrase had been with us for years, as if we were driving in a neighborhood where, if we made the right turn, we would meet the cure for Lyme disease.

In bed that night, I prayed: *May spirit shine light on all of Dana's physical problems and heal her. May she return to being a healthy twenty-year-old. May all this happen easily and for the good of all.* I focused my breath on this. I said this out loud. I imagined the joy I would feel. Yet I was frightened of what might be if the sonic treatments didn't work out. I worried about losing Dana. I worried about losing myself.

The second day, Dana went for a morning session while I shopped for food. This was the day she met Andrew. Ed had pushed Andrew's wheelchair into the treatment room and helped him into a recliner next to Dana. Even though he was listless, his head hanging to one side covered by the hood of his sweatshirt, he and Dana talked through the entire treatment, during which he disclosed that he was fighting cancer.

Until then, Dana had always been the sickest patient wherever we'd been. This was the first time she'd met someone close to her age who was more dangerously ill than she. At the end of the session, Andrew was able to hold his head up; he'd had miraculous results. We returned to the hotel, and Dana went on and on about Andrew. She identified with him. They were two young people dealing with the possibility of death.

When we went back the morning of the third day, Dana went in for her treatment and I hung out with Ed. He was a paunchy man who prided himself on his recent weight loss. He told me he was married to a young Asian woman who performed the "wifely duties" of ordering his home. It was more than I wanted to know.

"You're fit and slim," he observed. "I've lost a few pounds on a cleanse, but it's hard. How do you do it?"

"I have a yoga practice," I said, feeling annoyed.

In spite of Ed's personal disclosures and inappropriate attention, I was fascinated by the story about how he stumbled on this technology while working for the military. Back then he developed sonar devices for submarines. One day an elderly man happened to be standing next to him at the dock while he was testing his sonar equipment in the water. The elderly man stayed awhile chatting to Ed and began to "feel his legs buzzing." Later he experienced relief of his arthritic condition, so much so that he was able to walk free of pain.

Ed began his research with the elderly man. He would cart his machine to the man's house and treat him with different frequencies for varying amounts of time. He documented everything. Ed went on to partner with a university research department, where he began testing the effects of low-frequency "acoustic waveforms" on patients with vascular disease and osteoarthritis. His device was able to increase blood circulation, mobility, and range of motion, and reduce inflammation.

Ed had found that people with Lyme disease were unpredictable—some got positive results, some did not. Most felt worse before they got better. Back at home Dana just felt worse. We assumed she needed more treatments to get through this period of achiness, like Amber did. I committed to driving her to Las Vegas every two to three weeks for treatments for as long as it took for her to "turn the corner."

Dana stayed in touch with Andrew daily. Her relationship with him was private, a place where she could share herself more fully, explore her inner fears with someone who was equally challenged, and feel safe. I imagined she shared with him in a way she couldn't with me. With Andrew, perhaps she could dig into the dark side. I was relieved that she had a friend to really talk to. Very few of her school friends had stuck around for the hard stuff.

I asked her if she liked him, but she told me, "He's just a friend." *Do they give each other hope?* He was special to her because he understood what it was like to be different from everyone else in school. He knew about living with a serious health challenge. His seemed even more life threatening than hers, and for once, Dana was worried about someone other than herself.

Even though she hadn't had relief from her pain and swelling or any sign of improvement, we went to Las Vegas for the second series of treatments.

When we arrived, Ed asked, "Has anything changed since you were here last time?"

"Yes, Dana's new Lyme doctor, Dr. Loan, has started her on a simple oral antibiotic, azithromycin."

Ed was afraid this would mess up his research, but I found out later that day that there were other Lyme patients on antibiotics who were receiving his treatments. While I waited for Dana, I sat with Eileen, a round midwestern woman in her fifties, whose husband, Jim, also on antibiotics, was getting a treatment. She and I sat by the window facing a large treeless boulevard, and as I watched a feeble old woman inching down the sidewalk with her white Chihuahua, I listened to Eileen talk on and on in her lulling Southern voice.

"Well, it's gone on a loooong time now. Jim just lies in the recliner all day with the door closed, and sleeps in it at night. I don't know what to do. I take care of him and run our business too. I'm exhausted."

The next day Eileen and Jim rolled in a few minutes after us, and Eileen reported with triumph, "He's already feeling better. We took a short walk this morning." Great news for them, but I had a hard time expressing my enthusiasm for Jim's recovery since Dana was still swollen and achy. Eileen called me two weeks later and left a happy voice mail message: "Jim has improved and is back at work!" I didn't return her call.

One morning several weeks later, Dana ran into my bedroom completely hysterical, screaming that she'd just gotten a text from Andrew saying he had woken up in a pool of his own blood. Afraid to breathe, all I could think was, *What will Dana do if something bad happens to Andrew?* I didn't know if I could hold her up.

She paced, her face wincing and her skin white. "I told him I would be there for him! I told him I would come see him if things got worse. I have to go right away!"

"Okay. Let's figure this out—"

"I'm waiting to hear back from him about staying at his house."

Dana's relationship with Andrew existed in a bubble. I didn't know his parents or anything about him, and they didn't know me. She didn't know anyone in Andrew's life and he didn't know anyone in hers. Their bubble was not attached to the real world. It seemed she needed to see Andrew, as if this would somehow keep her alive.

"I have to go visit him. It could be the last time I see him. I have to go by myself. I'm leaving tomorrow first thing."

"Honey, you can't go by yourself. You're not well enough to drive!"

"Mom, I have to." With that she raced out of my bedroom and locked herself in the bathroom.

There's no way I'm letting her go!

An hour later Dana found me in the kitchen systematically chopping vegetables. I'd learned to keep my emotional responses on an even keel because any stress would set off a physical reaction in Dana's system. Rashes broke out and swelling increased. I couldn't bear to be the cause of any further discomfort. It was like I was wearing an internal girdle cinching my gut together so emotions wouldn't escape through my mouth. Dana couldn't even tolerate my rare, brief moments of joy, laughing, dancing, or singing. Her nervous system was a live wire.

"Mom, I'm going to stay with Andrew."

Oh my God. She's really going to do this. I felt I might actually split in two in front of her. Part of me would never feel right letting her do this, and part of me *wanted* her to take charge, to be independent. I thought this might be a good opportunity for her to take responsibility for herself, but it also felt like she'd be walking a tightrope with no safety net.

"Would you like me to go with you?"

"No, I want to go by myself. I'll go for some sonic treatments while I'm there."

"Oh. Okay."

I was spinning. I didn't know how to think about this. She was taking responsibility for her treatments, definitely a good thing but maybe also a bribe.

"I'm going to pack. Can you get the black suitcase for me?"

"Yes," I said, not wanting to cause a scene.

I desperately wanted her to be capable of driving out of town to visit a friend like a normal twenty-year-old, but I knew she was suffering from many symptoms that could make driving dangerous. I needed a break, but at the same time I was terrified. An image ran through my mind: Dana behind the wheel, pushing eighty miles per hour on the freeway for four and a half hours, her head pounding, exhausted. Would she be capable of making good decisions? Maybe Andrew was near death. I couldn't know what might happen, or control it. In my mind I severed the sinewy umbilical cord still connecting us. I got the suitcase.

"You must promise me you'll stop driving if you don't feel awake or aren't able to think clearly. And stay within the speed limit."

Dana nodded her head. She needed her freedom.

After she left, I began with the little things. I closed a door and let it make a sound. (When Dana was home and not in the sanctuary of her soundproof area, silence was mandatory. I had to turn the door handle all the way open, hold it while I closed it slowly, then gently, seamlessly, silently lift the handle back up to catch the latch.) In that brief moment of freedom from the tyranny of Dana's illness, I'd forgotten that the door wouldn't actually slam because all the doorjambs had foam weather stripping stuck to them to prevent the clang of wood against wood. I moved on to bigger things. I walked down the hall to my old sanctuary, the dance studio. I peeled off my sweatshirt and moved slowly at first, then furiously to Adele blasting "Rolling in the Deep."

I was twirling, running, gliding, and rolling on the floor. I strutted gracefully across the room on my toes, catching my reflection in the mirrors. I flew back across the floor in big leaps with my hands making fists in the air. I whipped fast ballet turns, eyes focused on the wall in front of me. When I reached the wall, I pushed hard against it. As arms flew up with hands flat, I fell forward, my weight pulling me as I crouched and then slipped down to my knees. I folded into a tight fetal ball.

In the late afternoon that same day, my phone rang; Dana was crying. She'd arrived at Andrew's house safely but had left her wallet in a gas station bathroom in Las Vegas when she stopped for gas. She had no driver's license, debit card, or money. I spoke quietly with her, forcing myself to sound non-judgmental, while inside I churned.

"Are *you* okay?"

"Yes."

"All right, just rest from the drive. I'll get back to you after I've made some calls. You should contact the gas station. See if someone found your wallet and turned it in. Don't worry, we'll figure this out."

I called a Wells Fargo branch in Las Vegas and explained the situation. I set up a meeting with a bank associate in Los Angeles who validated my identity. Dana would be able to pick up her new debit card the next day. I called the DMV but did not get through. Dana was in Nevada, not California, and I wasn't sure what to do. I was flooded with guilt. I'd needed a break. I hadn't *wanted* to go with her.

Andrew didn't live with his own family. He was staying with family friends who owned a hospital bed and were home during the day, so they could take care of him. Dana told me she was sleeping on the couch in this home and that his parents visited every night. Andrew was better than she'd thought. The night he texted her, he'd had a bad nose bleed. She learned he'd been sick for only one year, and before that he played on the varsity football team. He showed her a photo of himself looking healthy and muscular in his football uniform. His friends visited, even his old girlfriend.

Dana stayed with Andrew for three days, and when she returned home, she told me, "I'm not the only one who's there for him. He has a lot of friends who visit. I felt out of place." She wanted to be Andrew's savior. Her sadness and disappointment were only made worse by the fact that the sonic treatments weren't making her feel any better. A month later, sometime in July, Andrew stopped responding to her texts. She never heard from him again, never went back to Las Vegas, and never had another sonic treatment.

CHAPTER FIFTEEN

I'm Going to Heal Here

*Fate is like a strange, unpopular restaurant filled
with odd little waiters who bring you things you
never asked for and don't always like.*

— Lemony Snicket

In June 2011, right after Dana's last "sonic boom" session, I
sold our suburban home in Northridge. Both girls had finished high school and I was downsizing. Leaving the city
behind, we moved up to the small mountain community of
Topanga, California, into a hillside home that resembled a
redwood chalet.

"I'm going to heal here!" Dana announced after settling
into her new bedroom.

A month before we moved, Dana had started seeing Dr.
Loan, a Lyme Literate Medical Doctor (LLMD), who had a
new practice in Los Angeles and would be able to see Dana
once a month. After the first appointment with Dr. Loan, Dana

and I both decided that it was finally time for her to try the Lyme doctors' treatment of choice for chronic Lyme: intravenous (IV) antibiotics. It was an aggressive and controversial treatment used only by LLMDs. I'd never wanted to subject Dana to this potentially dangerous treatment, but at this point we needed something that would treat the deep infections, even if it meant going back to pharmaceuticals.

Dr. Loan used the most current protocols for the eradication of Lyme disease: a combination of IV antibiotics, other pharmaceuticals, and nutritional supplements to target specific symptoms directly. When we arrived at her office for Dana's second visit, the beautiful, sylphlike Dr. Loan welcomed Dana: "Hi, sweetie, how're you doing?"

Although Dana was pale and weak, I could see she was heartened by Dr. Loan's warm reception. I instantly lapsed into fantasy: *We're at a dance class and this is a friend's mom greeting Dana. Life is good and we're having a normal day.*

I was jarred back to reality as I heard Dana answer, "I'm feeling pretty bad. I think I want to start the IV treatment as soon as possible."

Dr. Loan proceeded to test her thoroughly. She touched Dana's face and looked into her eyes with a little light. She then assessed Dana's balance by asking her to walk across the room and back. I hoped her detective work would reveal all the reasons why she had not recovered. I imagined this as our last stop, that Dana's long illness would be cured here. I let the soothing voice of the doctor soak into me.

Dr. Loan spent a grueling two hours going over each of Dana's symptoms. We descended into the minutiae of the disease. Lyme doctors based their treatment on symptoms: what they were, how they changed, how often they arose, and how severe they were. Dana looked more and more pale and listless as the minutes crawled by. We left Dr. Loan's office with an exhaustive list of medicines for every symptom, as well as the prescription for IV antibiotics.

DANA'S DAILY MEDICINES AND SUPPLEMENTS

Antibacterial and Antiviral: IV Zithromax, IV Rocephin, rifampin, A-Bart, A-Bab, colloidal silver, Lauricidin

Pain: Advil, Aleve, ibuprofen

Hormones: Bioidentical thyroid, estradiol cream

Vitamins: B-12 injections, multivitamins, vitamin C, vitamin D, vitamin B6, vitamin E, iron, folic acid

Probiotics: VSL#3, Saccharomyces boulardii, custom probiotics

Mood: Lithium orotate

Binders: Chlorella, glucomannan, charcoal

Yeast: Amazon A-F, nystatin

Immune: Minerals: zinc, molybdenum, NT Factor Energy, Transfer Factor Multi-Immune, resveratrol, selenium, Immune Renew

Inflammation: Carlson's Omega, Opti-Magnesium

Adrenal Support: Adrenal Essence, Forskolin, ActiFolate, pantothenic acid

Liver/Gall Bladder Support: IV glutathione, oral glutathione, Systemic Formulas Lb Liver/Gall Bladder, Ultra Liver Support, Actigall

Herx Die-Off (reaction to killing bacteria): Pectasol-C, Alkabase, Alka Gold, Advil, warm water and lemon, quercetin

Sinus: Phosphatidylcholine, Pycnogenol, Arginine, Ornithine

Lymphatic: Lymphomyosot, L-Drain, K-Drain, Pekana Itires cream

Gut: DGL, Gastric Repair, Intestinal Repair, Aloe Ferox, proteolytic enzymes, Allergy Research Group Pancreas, Digest

Detox: Neuro-Antitox II Basic, Medcaps DPO, IMN-V II, Colace

Eye: Erythromycin ointment

Back at home I sat at my desk reading the long list of medications, like a runaway roll of toilet paper. I was responsible for researching where to purchase the drugs for the best price and obtaining them as soon as possible. I mentally repeated the names of the drugs again and again, memorizing them, befriending them, normalizing them. Anxiety rose in my belly, and my mouth watered. I felt my life being torn into the tiniest pieces. I stood up, faced the large window that looked out into my garden, and yelled, "We *are* going to do this!" This treatment would be my new religion.

I spent hours on the internet and phone procuring Dana's meds. I trudged around the confines of the chalet. I had no other life. I typed up a detailed schedule with the days and times each medication was to be taken, and carefully noted dosages. I marked the calendar with the dates that each of the medicines would run out. These schedules haunted me. It would be my fault if Dana didn't take the right medicine or got the wrong dosage or didn't have what she needed. The living room became a pharmacy. I bought a small white cabinet and placed it next to the couch to conceal the mountain of supplies.

Dana had a port surgically inserted into her left arm so we could administer the IV antibiotics at home. The procedure should have taken one hour but took three, and produced pain in the left side of her chest where the internal line was threaded inside a blood vessel from her arm into her chest. Several days after the port was inserted, Dana's nurse, Susan, came to our house to start the IV treatments. She taught her how to hook up the IV bag tubing to the short line on the outside of her arm at the port site. When Dana wasn't using the line, she would disconnect the IV bag and wrap her left arm to protect the short protruding line.

Once a week I had to change the needle at the port site. Changing the needle weekly decreased the risk of infection and gave Dana a break, for a few hours to a few days, depending on the IV schedule, from having a line continuously outside her arm. I was nervous poking the thick needle through her tender skin each week, attempting to get it in the right spot so I didn't cause bleeding. It was a job I never wanted, but for my daughter I would do anything. I was less expensive than hiring a regular home care nurse. Eventually, Dana became her own nurse and I her assistant. Living in our new home, we ran a small medical facility for one.

I snuck out to Whole Foods after dinner one night while Dana was glued to her computer watching a documentary. Inside the double glass doors I found more than simple nourishment. I made my way to the massage chair to have my back lovingly kneaded. I couldn't wait to settle my face in the circular head cradle, close my eyes, and let Nancy lighten my burden for a few minutes. After the massage I stayed flopped on the bent chair with my face in the cradle, drifting off into memories of happier times.

I met William at Whole Foods in January 2007, two weeks before Dana got sick. Bent over the vegetable case examining lettuce, I was choosing between the romaine and baby greens when I felt a tap on my shoulder. I swung around and looked up at a stunning face. He was tall, dark-skinned, gorgeous, and smiling.

"Do I know you?"

I looked into his eyes and clearly saw he was talking to me.

"I don't think so."

"*Could* I know you?" he asked in a singsongy way. I could hear it now like music playing.

I was bowled over by his clear face and tight body. I couldn't believe he was talking to me. *Is it the spandex pants that hug my buns?* I was terribly unnerved by his overture. He handed me his card, and I noted he was a physical trainer. I gave him my cell number. *That's safe, isn't it?* He looked thirty-five years old to my fifty-four. I proceeded to shop until I was out of his sight, then raced down the aisle to check out. I had to get out of there. What if he tried to talk to me again? I got on the freeway heading home and my phone rang.

"I thought I would say good-bye to you at the checkout, but you were gone already."

"Yep."

"Can I take you to dinner sometime soon?"

"Umm. That would be lovely. I'm free next weekend."

"How is next Saturday night at seven?"

A real date.

I started sneaking out at night after my teenage daughters were asleep. William would meet me at my car and walk me into his apartment building with his arm securely wrapped around my shoulders.

"How are you, my beautiful rose? You look sexy in those jeans."

Before we could get into his apartment, William would grab me, run his hands down my back, caressing me, while fixing me with his eyes. He took his time, touching me with gentle passion, while I danced with him, wide open. Entwined with him, I was tousled, sweaty, wrung out, and joyous.

Dana got sick two weeks after I met William, and soon after, her illness prevented me from leaving the house. Though I already knew he wasn't going to be the one I would grow old with, he was the one I called late at night to get the worry and confusion off my chest. Eventually, what was left of our relationship faded as Dana's illness took over my life.

After my massage I cruised the food aisles to pick up olive oil, almond butter, gluten-free granola, and other items. Seeing the same items every time, all stacked neatly on their shelves where they were supposed to be, made me feel peaceful. There was no order like this in my life. I was the last customer in the checkout line, actually the last customer in the store. I wanted to stay in this ordered, abundant universe as long as possible. Two of the young guys at the cash register who saw me here almost every day began to serenade me as they sang along with the music playing over the PA system: the Four Tops, "Reach Out, I'll Be There."

Their healthy exuberance brought tears to my eyes as I paid for my groceries and danced my way out of the store with a full bag.

CHAPTER SIXTEEN

Living the IV Life

*It's all right if you grow your wings
on the way down.*

— Robert Bly

Perched on a hill, surrounded by old, healthy oak trees, our new home was like a tree house. The entire third floor was my bedroom. It had rich rosewood flooring, a trestle-beamed ceiling, and eight-foot-high windows opening into the treetops. It was the lightest part of the house. My sanctuary. I got to know whole tree branches as if they were my own limbs. Sleeping among the trees rejuvenated me enough to get through the next day. Sunrise greeted me beaming in through tall curtainless windows—a glorious way to wake up!

Then one less than glorious morning, I heard in my dream: "Mommeeee!"

Moments after jerking awake, the feeling of dread shocked me from the inside. My daughter was in pain somewhere in the house.

"Mommeeee!"

I raced down the stairs to help her.

What's the crisis? Is her breathing bad? Has the gardener's exhaust from the blowers gotten into the house from a window I left open? Is her blackout shade angled, letting in bright flecks of light?

As I skidded onto the landing, I heard her accusing voice: "What's that smell? It's hurting my head!"

I saw the open window in the hallway and smelled the exhaust. My heart sank. I couldn't stop her pain. I felt like punching my hand through the window. Instead, I shut it hard and grabbed the peppermint spray bottle that we left out for just this reason. I sprayed the air like a maniac. I sprayed until she stopped yelling. I sprayed until my hand went numb.

On another morning, when Dana was extremely weak, she climbed up the narrow wood staircase to use my bathroom. Her own bathroom downstairs had a bad smell, like a rat had died in the wall. It was early and she was achy, wearing only a towel wrapped around her waist. Clothes bothered her. I heard her brush her teeth, and when she came out of the bathroom, she stopped to pet our cat Betty, asleep on my bed.

She didn't say "good morning" to me; she just headed down the stairs. As I drifted back to sleep, a thunderous sound, like a chimney collapsing, jolted me awake. My heart jumped out of my chest. Time slowed. It took me forever to get out of bed and run. I stood at the top of the stairs, riveted; Dana was slumped in a heap on the stone floor at the bottom of the stairs. I was with her in my next breath. *After all the years of saving her life, will she die of an accident tripping on her towel?* I bent over and listened for her breath. She giggled. *She's alive!*

As I held Dana in my arms on the landing, I remembered the fluffy white bunny I'd had when I was seven. My sisters and I carried her around upside down, with her little legs sticking up. We fed her and played with her, but after a month she died. I always thought we killed her by carrying her upside down.

⁕

Our day began when Dana awoke around 10:00 a.m., groggy, achy, and not wanting to talk. She tromped down the wood stairs to the ground floor and shuffled into the kitchen to make her breakfast of sautéed greens and poached eggs. Years before, she dined on pancakes like other kids. Now her stomach hurt if she ate grains. It was sometimes hard to tell what hurt her stomach since a large part of what she ingested consisted of handfuls of supplements and pharmaceutical meds.

I stepped carefully down two flights of stairs, carrying her bulky eleven-pound air purifier, which ran all day in the living room, filtering irritants from the air Dana breathed. Sleep-walking through the routine I loathed, I thought about how our lives had become so laborious. There was little enjoyment. Each day was made up of a series of tasks meant to treat the monster Lyme disease. It was exhausting, but I had to override my loathing and make our days into a lighthearted routine, so we could pretend wellness was on its way.

Down in the basement laundry, each dirty, sweaty garment of Dana's passed through my hands on its way into the washer. I poured in a small amount of no-phosphate detergent and fifteen drops of eucalyptus oil to mask the odor. I folded each shirt, pair of pants, dress, and undergarment, noting which ones I had a distaste for. The ones shredding, formless, and soft from too much wear were my least favorite. Dana's swelling made it impossible for her to put on fitted clothes, so she wore the same stretched-out clothing day after day.

I had a particular dislike for the faded purple leggings, bought during the second year of Dana's illness. These had become her go-to pants for comfort. Part of me cleaned, folded, and ordered her belongings to bring tidiness to the chaos, while part of me wanted to burn them to ash and bury them far beneath the earth. *Am I going to be okay if Dana dies?* I folded the laundry. I put the clothes away.

I watched Dana take a vitamin B12 syringe out of the refrigerator and inject herself on her multibruised backside. Settling on the living room couch, she skillfully hooked her arm up to the IV bag and hung the bag on the pole. She then placed an oxygen cannula in her nose so she could inhale pure oxygen from the generator to support her labored breathing.

An hour later she swallowed the prescription medications that had to be taken *without* food while I prepared her special enema coffee, a blend of green coffees "finely ground," ordered from Canada. I cooled the simmered coffee down in the freezer so it was still warm but not too warm, or it would burn her insides. We knew this because it happened once and took a week for her to recover. Thinking about all the treatments—the ones that were ingested orally, injected directly into her bloodstream, injected intramuscularly, and inserted rectally—made my teeth clench so forcibly it became hard to swallow. I struggled to keep from screaming, which would cause Dana even more pain. *How is it possible for a young person to endure this?*

⁕ ⁕ ⁕ ⁕ ⁑ ⁕ ⁕ ⁕ ⁕

One day I left for an hour to press my anger into the Pilates machine, my weekly escape. I passed old trees with leaves turning yellow, ready to fall. I thought about how I was in love with the canyon as I wound down the road. I parked at Pine Tree Circle, the town center. My instructor, Nannette, would take me through a Pilates workout to exercise my muscles, build core strength, and remind me of my body's innate health. I was in training for my life.

"Hi, Nannette."

"Hello, Anna. How's your daughter?"

"Not good, she's more swollen. Work me hard today—I need to forget for an hour. Let's do abs and butt-burner."

"Okay, lady! You asked for it. I'll warm up your legs and upper body, then we'll do a set of butt-building leg exercises lying on your side. Want to finish with the jump board?"

"Yeah. Now you're talking!"

I escaped to a world away from my home, where I had one hour to release my frustration and recuperate. Nannette pounded her fists into my gluteal muscles after I did butt-burner. I was just beginning to let go of tension when the ring of my pink-and-white cell phone pierced the mood. I saw it was Dana calling and, in spite of my reluctance to have my sacred hour interrupted, I answered reflexively.

"Momma, I just did something wrong and my chest hurts and it's hard to breathe!"

Suppressing alarm, I asked, "What happened?"

"I forgot to fill the line before I inserted my IV, and I got air in my line."

"Okay, okay, I am sure it's okay. Let me call your nurse."

"It says on the internet that you should get to an emergency room because you could have an embolism!"

"I'll call you right back."

I sat up on the Pilates machine, my phone pressed tightly against my pale face, anxiously waiting for the nurse to answer. "Philippe, Dana just did her IV without filling the line first. Do I need to take her to the emergency room?" My heart beat so hard it vibrated my body. He reassured me that she would be fine.

I called Dana back. "Honey, Philippe says you'll be fine."

"But it's still hard to breathe."

"Philippe said your port has a filter and you can't have an embolism. Don't be scared—it will pass and you'll be fine. Please relax until I get home."

I resumed my Pilates session, my momentary escape. My body moved with difficulty in the foot straps. I was no longer there.

When I returned home, I clipped a tiny, pink Double Delight rose from my garden. I slipped it into a small glass vase and sat it on the mantel across from Dana. Her middle name is Rose. She responded sweetly. "Thanks, Momma. These are my favorite! Let me smell it." I was still coming down from the scare. Dana too—she looked drained of color.

As Dana showered, I chopped vegetables into small squares and started cooking her lunch. She ate only steamed vegetables, chicken, fish, and grass-fed beef. She didn't eat dairy, soy, nuts, grains, sugar, or anything else that caused inflammation and bloating. Dana came into the kitchen with her hair wrapped in a towel. The near disaster from earlier in the day was almost forgotten. She ate her lunch and downed the supplements that had to be taken *with* food.

After lunch Dana lay back on the couch and hooked up the next IV. To amuse herself, she stacked all her bottles and jars of medicine in a towering sculpture on the oval coffee table. She looked so tiny behind the sculpture. The antibiotic dripped slowly into her arm for an hour and a half. All the while Dana intently watched documentaries on her computer, educating herself about various environmental disasters like water contamination and strip mining, and their effect on the health of local residents.

I thought about the connection between environmental toxins and toxic infections as I filled the ionic foot spa with warm water to soak Dana's feet for thirty minutes while we watched the videos together. Her doctor had encouraged her to use the foot spa as a method to remove toxins and heavy metals from her body. The routine of endless tasks required to keep Dana's body functioning had me operating on automatic. Her voice cut through my blankness.

"I don't feel like I'm here. I'm not myself, Momma."

"What do you mean?"

"I keep thinking that I don't want to be here. I'm so depressed."

"You're definitely feeling the results of your head pain. Are you suicidal?"

"I'm not, Momma."

Behind my placid façade was a raging river of panic. I appeared serene and efficient on the outside, like the still surface of a river before it plunges over a cliff and becomes nothing but churning foam. Even though my twenty-two-year practice of Kundalini Yoga had cultivated balance in my breath and body, I was desecrated by sorrow.

When Dana finished soaking her feet, I wandered outside to water my flowers, but instead sank into the muslin hammock hanging in the garden. I smelled lavender. My muscles went limp. I succumbed to the crying in my heart. I listened to the trees rustling, the birds singing to each other. The hammock cradled me and rocked me gently.

That evening I finally had a chance to relax in the bath with a book. I filled the tub with warm, silky water, adding the aroma of lavender oil.

"Mommy!" Dana's voice ripped through me.

Like I had a thousand times before, I saw the emergency room looming before me. I jumped out of the bath, seized a towel, and dashed, my hair dripping water, down two flights of stairs, while inside I raged at Dana for shattering my peace.

"Mom, the two packets of seeds I ordered on the internet are fresh, not dried like I thought. They have to be planted right away."

I checked my internal screaming so I could respond without attacking her.

"Okay."

"What did you put on your hair? You smell!"

I raised my hands up in a gesture of surrender and forced a smile.

"And there's another thing. I feel stupid, but these two are supposed to be germinated in spring." She held up the two packets of seeds for me to see.

"Oh! Do you think we can trick them because we live in the temperate climate of California?"

"We can't wait till spring. Do we have potting soil?"

"I have a couple of pots with soil in them that you could start with." I looked at the clock on the wall and added, "Since it's eight at night and nothing's open." We were always losing track of time.

"All right! Let's go outside."

In spite of myself, Dana's enthusiasm was irresistible and I couldn't help but participate. Gardens had been around me all my life. When I was a child, my father dug up one side of our driveway and planted an exotic garden. During my parents' travels all over the world, he clipped cuttings from foliage he loved and smuggled them home in his suitcase to plant in his beloved driveway garden. We had the only Mexican cherimoya tree in the neighborhood. Our blossoming, fragrant Hawaiian plumerias looked gorgeous in the spring and like stubs in the fall and winter.

My children spent hours with Papa in his garden when they were little. He introduced them to tropical fruits such as guavas, star fruit, kumquats, and papayas. Years ago, when Papa died suddenly, my girls and I made a ceramic sign, "Papa's Memorial Garden," and planted it in our yard with vegetables we could harvest and eat. We took this handmade sign with us to our new rented house in the mountains and hung it over our raised-bed vegetable garden.

I put on sweats and joined Dana on the front patio.

Reading from the packet of seeds, she explained: "It does not like to be transplanted and likes dry soil. Neem is a tree."

"A tree? That we have to plant for a lifetime at our rented house? I thought this was a vegetable garden, not a forest!"

Giggling, Dana took out one of the seeds.

"I went a little overboard when I ordered these medicinal seeds online. They need to be planted in warm soil with good drainage. We can use my bed mat to heat the seeds from underneath!"

"I hardly think so—too expensive to turn on twenty-four/seven for three weeks just to keep a small pot of soil warm. I vote we put the pot in the little TV room that gets sunshine through the windows."

"Yeah, that's a good place for it, like an indoor greenhouse. And then there's the goldenseal. It needs to be planted in a shade garden with two inches deep of leaf mulch."

"Okay. Let's plant it now and gather leaves this week. It won't take long 'cause it's fall!"

This glorious fun lasted all of fifteen minutes before Dana's energy plummeted. Crabby and tired again, she plopped on the couch and wanted me out of the room. I was eager for those fifteen minutes of sharing something she had her heart set on. I went from black and white to Technicolor. I smiled until my mouth hurt. In those fifteen minutes she projected the illusion of being well.

One morning I was putting Dana's weekly needle in the port in her arm, but blood was not flowing through the line. Something was wrong. I poked her six times, finally thinking I'd managed to get the needle into the port. When we hooked up the IV antibiotics, her arm swelled up to the size of a mango, indicating that the needle was not in the port, so we called in a nurse who was able to properly insert the needle.

The next day we went to the hospital to have the port examined. Dana had been practicing "bound lotus," a yoga pose practitioners believed could cure any ailment. She had been sitting in this position, with her arms crossed behind her back holding on to her feet from their cross-legged position in front, for twenty minutes every day. This position had caused her ribs to press on the port, which changed the angle of entry. Fortunately, it did not require surgery; I just had to hold it level when I inserted the needle from then on.

The pine-resin salve slathering began four days later. This sticky substance was applied all over Dana's body before bedtime. The salve, made of olive oil and tree saps, was claimed to rejuvenate skin and draw out toxins. She was ready to find out if she could get her swelling down by using the salve. When she did, she became even more tired and spacey, and believed this was a good thing because it proved the medicine was working. She used up a jar of the salve twice a week, so we invested in fifteen jars and got a wholesale price. Her sheets turned translucent yellow. I hoped, like I did with every treatment, that just maybe this treatment, by going where all other treatments had failed to go, would cause a massive internal genocide of the Lyme bacteria.

It seemed there wasn't anything Dana wouldn't try to help herself get well. Following the failure of the bound lotus experiment, she sheepishly informed me one morning that two of her Lyme friends had been drinking their pee and feeling better! *Oh boy.* I'd heard of urine therapy. I was not shocked; however, I shuddered at the lengths Dana continued to go to. Moved actually, almost to tears. The next day she came into the kitchen with a small glass about a third full of reddish clear liquid.

"Is that what I think it is?"

"Yes."

"Is the red color from your B12?"

"I don't know."

"Ohhhh. Well, cheers! Would you like to add water? How about some honey?"

"Ewww."

I listened to her footsteps and the slam of the bathroom door, then I heard a loud groan. She resurfaced and I hugged her. She'd done it!

This went on once a day for a week until Dr. Loan told us that the red color in Dana's urine was from her rifampin antibiotic. We figured that it wasn't good for her to "recycle" the antibiotic, so Dana's brave experiment with urine therapy was now officially over.

⁕ ⁕ ⁕

We sat at midnight chatting, as we did most evenings when Dana could tolerate my company.

"I am going on a date tomorrow."

"Really? I haven't seen you leave the living room in weeks."

"I don't feel great, but I do feel a little better and I'm bored. I want to get out of the house."

"That's a good sign!"

"Maybe being off the antibiotics for a few days has helped my body calm down."

After Dana had taken the IV antibiotics full time for four months, Dr. Loan decided she should try the new protocol of "pulsing" her IV Rocephin—four days on, three days off. It was something new the Lyme doctors were trying. Dr. Loan agreed to let her try it in an attempt to alleviate the severe side effects she'd been experiencing from the antibiotics. Pulsing was supposed to give her body a break—and trick the bacteria into coming out of hiding so they would be more vulnerable to the next round of antibiotics.

"I'm feeling a little pressure about the date," Dana confided. "It takes me so long to get ready. I'll have to get up early, around ten, then take my medicine, eat, lie on the magnet, eat, take medicine, and shower. It'll take me an hour to dry my hair and put on my makeup. All just to get out the door by seven p.m."

"Wow, a whole day just to prepare for your date. Maybe you could wash your hair tonight?"

"No, 'cause then I have to sleep on it and it won't look good. I'm exhausted thinking about all the things I'll have to do. Maybe I won't go out tomorrow."

"Look at you. Just *thinking* about doing something is too much!"

We fell off the couch, laughing hysterically.

CHAPTER SEVENTEEN

Firefall

In the end, just three things matter:
How well we have lived
How well we have loved
How well we have learned to let go.

— Jack Kornfield

Dana seemed to be feeling a little better on the new protocol, and I silently prepared myself to leave for a week, the first time in a year. I'd lost myself to the illness. Over the years I'd suppressed my enthusiasm, my pleasure, and my animated personality. I needed to reexperience my true self, away from the pressure cooker of Dana's discomfort. I intended to go guilt-free into my Yosemite vacation. *It is my human right to feel pleasure.* At home there was so much pain. I was not sure I would remember how to be social, but I planned to hike till I was wrung out, eat tasty gourmet food, and laugh from my belly again.

I landed at the Oakland airport, where my sister Jain and her husband, Steven, picked me up and drove me to their big white house in the Berkeley Hills. It was grand and sophisticated, with a view of the San Francisco Bay. My sister took good care of me. My room was cozy and welcoming, the guest bed made with fresh, crisp sheets. I stretched out on the down comforter, my eyes glazing over with grateful tears.

That night we dined at a wonderful fish restaurant, and when we settled into our seats, Jain exclaimed, "So, you're going back to Yosemite! Remember when Dad took us there? All I remember is how we argued in the car during the long drive, and that you found an arrowhead on a hike."

"Yeah, I remember that! You tried to steal it!"

Jain laughed.

It was all coming back to me and I asked, "Do you remember the weird, round hollows in a granite boulder by our campsite?"

"No."

"They were made by Native Americans, and I loved running my hands into the smooth bowls. It's where they ground their acorns—I could almost feel the flour for their bread. I'm excited to go back!"

In the morning Jain and Steven drove me into San Francisco. Like parents dropping their child off for a class camping trip, they wouldn't leave until they saw my luggage loaded on the bus to Yosemite. Steven pulled me aside and whispered in my ear that he noticed some good-looking men boarding the bus. I decided then and there that I was going to Yosemite without my story. I wouldn't mention my daughter's illness. I'd just be me. *But who am I if I'm not the heroic, long-suffering mother of a frightfully sick child?*

On our first morning, the handsome, thirtysomething guide, Sam, led fifteen of us up the Panorama Trail, which switchbacked steeply up the mountain, revealing views of Half Dome, Glacier Point, and the Yosemite Valley. I felt my heart peel open with every step. Even though my pack cut into my waist, I refused to stop. I refused to act like an old lady. I pushed myself to keep up with Sam, to get to the top. I laughed to myself as I remembered how Dad pushed us kids to just keep going, even when we begged to turn around. He would reassure us that the view would be worth the effort. He always wanted to scale the highest peak with the best view. That was his thing.

I navigated the rocky parts of the trail, keeping my eyes on the ever-changing expanse of granite peaks. It was rigorous, but inside I was singing. We lunched at the top, where pounding waters rippled off the granite cliffs, clearing everything from my mind. Just me on a rock with my sandwich and all of Yosemite Valley below. After eating, everyone gathered and descended sharply down the Mist Trail, stair stepping past unforgettable vistas. My legs were strong but rubbery from miles of downhill stepping. I was glorious, winded, and humming to myself as I absorbed the scenery, grateful for this opportunity to feel good again.

On the third night an early snow began to fall. I layered up my clothes and went outside to marvel at the heavenly landscape. Every leaf was touched by white powder, altering the scenery entirely from the day before when autumn had changed the colors. We were supposed to go to Tuolumne Meadows for a long hike the next day, but by morning the roads were closed due to heavy snowfall.

I was nine years old the last time I hiked in Yosemite. It was the middle of summer, and my father had enthusiastically taken us on yet another camping trip where we would be sleeping in sleeping bags and cooking on a campfire. We were city girls at home in Los Angeles, but as soon as we hit the trail, we became wilderness girls. One morning he took us to Tuolumne Meadows, where we walked around until we found a flat, shady place near a creek to eat our picnic lunch.

Dad laid out a blanket and Mom unpacked chips, pickles, and a can of tuna for each of us. She spotted wild scallions growing near the creek and showed us how to pull them out of the ground. I chopped mine into tiny pieces with my Girl Scout pocketknife and sprinkled them over the packed tuna, filling the can. The wild scallions were crunchy and fresh, making the fishy tuna taste more delicious than I could imagine. We sat in silence, savoring our lunch while we focused on the mountains rising over the meadow and listened to the music of the flowing water.

Our hiking group, mostly grown-up city kids and baby boomers, was not camping but staying at the grand and luxurious Ahwahnee Hotel, situated at the mouth of the Yosemite Valley, which was surrounded by glacier-carved stone mountains. The hotel's three rustic stories were constructed from river stones, timber, concrete, and glass, an architectural feat in the 1920s.

We were given a tour before dinner one night and got to see the Solarium on the grand floor, where natural light floods in through the two-story-high windows facing a view of majestic Glacier Point. Our tour guide told us that the room was built for the original owner's wife so she could stay warm while watching the famously spectacular Yosemite Firefall plunging over the cliffs, three thousand feet down to the valley floor. It turns out that the last Firefall was conducted in 1968. My family and I were there in 1962.

"Has anyone seen the Firefall?"

I saw the Firefall!

The guide saw my eyes light up and asked me directly if I had ever seen it. I nodded and he asked me to share my memory. It turns out that I was the only one in the room who'd had the privilege of witnessing this unusual spectacle!

"I was nine years old when my dad drove our old Ford station wagon, with our camping gear piled on top, into Yosemite. We were here for a week, and one night my parents told us kids if we got into our pajamas and brushed our teeth, they would take us on an adventure. We climbed in the car and drove up the mountain. When we got to the top, there was a crowd of people standing around a huge bonfire of red fir bark. It had a searing pine smell that went up my nose. We were completely entranced and the crowd was quiet, waiting with anticipation."

I looked into the faces of my audience and took a breath. They were rapt, so I continued sharing my experience.

"A voice from below shouted, 'Hello, Glacier!' Then the ranger yelled, 'Hello, Camp Curry!' The response was 'Let the fire fall!' Then the ranger grabbed a big shovel and heaved the coals over the precipice of Glacier Point. The red heat flowed over the cliff like a burning waterfall."

Seventeen pairs of eyes imagined this with me. Out of the periphery of my vision, I caught sight of the army-green Park Ranger shirt. He was thanking "Anna." *That's me!* What a feeling!

CHAPTER EIGHTEEN

Ancient Influences

*You can go other places, all right—you can live on the
other side of the world, but you can't ever leave home.*

— Sue Monk Kidd, *The Mermaid Chair*

In September 2011 Dana was still direly ill when Cayla traveled to Africa again, four months after graduating from college. She ventured to Senegal alone to train with her new mentor, Oumar, a master teacher of traditional West African dance and drumming. Oumar spoke English and had taken on the responsibility of looking after Cayla. She stayed in a small village where she lived in a family household of thirty people. Life in her village was communal, and family was all-important. When people asked about her own family, they couldn't believe that her sister had been ill for so long. Oumar wanted to help Cayla and arranged to take her to the most powerful medicine man in the village.

She called me a day later. "I have to tell you something. Oumar took me to see a medicine man named Elhadji. He's very old. He can help Dana. Oumar translated for me because I couldn't understand what he was saying in Wolof. He just kept looking at me with his deep eyes. We have to go back to see him again to get the medicinal bark for Dana. He's going to Goree Island to harvest it."

Two weeks later Cayla returned to visit the healer with Oumar. Elhadji handed Cayla the bark. It was for Dana *and* Cayla. Elhadji told her the medicine would heal her of her sadness and guilt if she drank it for one month and buried the remains in the earth. It could not be burned, or the remedy would not work. Cayla sipped her boiled bark potion every day, hoping it would diminish the pain of losing her sister to an illness.

Cayla sent Dana's bark to me wrapped in a paper bag with special instructions, describing exactly how it was to be boiled, and exactly how Dana was supposed to drink it if she expected to cure her illness. The natural cure came at a time when Dana was following an aggressive pharmaceutical protocol. It would be too dangerous to mix the two. I held the bag, my fingers entwined tightly around it, my tears soaking in. I placed it on my meditation altar. Maybe here the miracle could take place between medicines, between sisters, between cultures, between healing forces.

Not long after I received the medicinal bark, I sat peacefully in front of my altar, chanting as I have done daily for many years.

"Sa Ta Na Ma . . . Sa Ta Na Ma . . ." I intoned as I pressed each of my fingers in turn to my thumbs with each syllable of sound. I used this Kundalini Yoga meditation to calm my mind. I finished in silence, with my hands folded over my heart. My eyes opened and focused intensely on the bark from Senegal. The dark brown tree bark lay there in its place of honor on my altar, representing a confluence of worlds. Tiny pearls of sweat collected on my forehead; my palms became moist. I heard a woodpecker hammering on the side of the house, like a faucet dripping, incessant and irritating. The bark had unraveled something in my soul.

One day when I was seven, my mother and I were in her garage art studio. I sat at a little table, drawing a house. I didn't like it. It didn't look the way I wanted it to. I ripped the paper out of the coloring pad and crumpled it in my hands. My mother got up from her easel, walked over quietly, and picked up the discarded paper. Flattening it out, she said, "Make it into something else." *Oh, it can be something else!* This was new for me. It affected everything I saw. My mother had ways of expanding my perception of the world.

I was ten years old when my parents began to travel the world and bring back artifacts from other places. The first of these were two Mexican masks, made of dried straw, with eyeless faces and gaping mouths. My mother hung them on the wall facing the front door, where they scared unsuspecting guests. My mother was not fond of *ordinary*; she was an artist. Things had to challenge, provoke, or puzzle. My impressionable mind memorized the unfamiliar, ethnic forms scattered throughout our home until they became as much a part of me as everything else.

On the way to the living room, I had to walk under the colorful Indonesian masks made of real skin and hair, floating from invisible strands fastened to the ceiling. As I passed, I could hear the soft, sandy sound made by the hair as it moved. Their exaggerated expressions would catch my breath. They were wild and crazy, and I never wanted to touch them.

We lived in an old Spanish-style home in West Los Angeles. Its soft, earthy lines, arched doorways, tile floors, and fat, hand-painted wooden beams that held up the A-frame living room contrasted with the straight, modern lines of my mother's Danish teak furniture. Hanging on the wall near the Indonesian masks, a large canvas covered with my mother's thick knife strokes in oil paint depicted Degas-inspired ballet dancers in pink tutus. Her small, roughly molded bronze human figurines were displayed on the buffet.

My parents never traveled to Africa, but we had two wooden ceremonial African masks hanging above the hearth. My mother had seen them in an import store and had fallen in love. As a teenager I would sit on the bright orange couch in the living room, staring at the masks while listening to the Beatles "Do You Want To Know A Secret." I wondered what the masks would whisper to me if I got close enough. Would the wide forehead confer wisdom? Would the oversized mouth and chin lend me strength and determination? What kind of power could these masks impart? What would I become if I wore one?

I lifted one of the African masks off the wall. It was much lighter than I'd expected. The wood smelled like dust and sweat. I pressed it to my face, and as I looked through the eyeholes, I entered the unspeakable subtlety of the mask's power. For as long as I could remember, I saw vibrations that other people didn't see. I could lie down under a tree and see light energy rippling off its leaves, pulsing against the blue sky. I knew the masks carried energy. No one ever talked about what I could sense; no one talked about the different energies in our house. I wanted to learn from the masks. I had a sense that what they had to teach me was beyond what I knew of my family, my religion, and my culture.

I was raised in seasons punctuated by Jewish holiday celebrations. On my sacred thirteenth birthday, I entered womanhood chanting in Hebrew from a centuries-old Torah scroll made of real parchment. A record of me singing during my Bat Mitzvah service was kept in the stereo cabinet in the living room. Also in the living room, on top of the upright piano, was a three-foot-long ram's horn nestled in a crocheted orange, pink, and black shawl my grandmother had made. The ram's horn, a "shofar," was traditionally blown on the Jewish High Holy Days—an ancient call to awakening. It was difficult to play, but my sister Jain could pucker her lips and make a yelping elephant sound on it.

Purim, a Jewish holiday celebrated on the full moon of the spring equinox, was when we all wore costumes, including masks. I loved it because it was a crazy, joyous holiday with dancing, noise making, booing, cheering, singing, and shouting. Along with all the kids, I would wave my "grogger," a little metal case with loud gears inside that sounded like a motor grinding. I first experienced the power of putting on a "mask" during Purim when I impersonated the exquisite Queen Esther, who risked her life to save her people. When my mother applied makeup on my little girl face, I *became* the illustrious Queen Esther, graceful and persuasive, knowing what was best for her people. Being Esther, I felt I could conquer anything.

I sat with the Senegalese bark before me. It had me in a trance. I felt the medicine man and the indigenous tree who offered its skin. I heard Cayla's cries, a chorus of powerful prayers. Hope rose through my chest into my throat, where hushed sounds formed. I sang the gorgeous blessing for healing in Hebrew, the Mi Shebeyrach:

Mi Shebeirach avoteinu v'imoteinu, Avraham,
Yitzchak v'Yaakov, Sarah, Rivkah, Rachel v'Lei-ah,
hu y'vareich et hacholim. HaKadosh Baruch Hu
yimalei rachamim aleihem, l'hachalimam ul'rapo-
tam ul'hachazikam, v'yishlach lahem m'heirah r'fuah,
r'fuah shleimah min hashamayim, r'fuat hanefesh
ur'fuat haguf, hashta baagala uviz'man kariv.
V'nomar: Amen.

May the one who blessed our ancestors, Abraham, Isaac and Jacob, Sarah, Rebecca, Rachel and Leah, bless and heal those who are ill. May the Blessed Holy One be filled with compassion for their health to be restored and their strength to be revived. May God swiftly send them a complete renewal of body and spirit, and let us say, Amen.

CHAPTER NINETEEN

Thanksgiving 2011

*I am grateful for what I am and have. My thanksgiving
is perpetual. It is surprising how contented one can be
with nothing definite—only a sense of existence.*

— Henry David Thoreau

A handmade weaving hung on the wall near the front door
of our Topanga mountain chalet. It was about three and a
half feet wide by five feet tall and had been woven by the hands
of my family eleven years before at a Thanksgiving reunion.
Back then, we all stood together chatting, laughing, and weaving
fabric strips, photos, and other personal items into the loom
I had created from driftwood and rope. In the cross weave
were remnants of Cayla's favorite old shorts, my mother's army-
green wool sweater, one of my father's T-shirts, fake zebra fur,
shiny gold spandex, and purple quilted cotton.

Cayla and Dana glued little beach stones they had collected onto the wooden frame. My sister Tovya tied a piece of

turquoise sea glass to a strand of green raffia and attached it to the warp. A photo of me and my sister Jain posing at the beach, looking identical with our long blond hair and big round sunglasses, dangled on a red ribbon tied to the frame. My mother forgot to bring something personal to add, so she took off her sweater, cut it into strips, and wove it in. The circular ribbed collar hung like a necklace, with a photo of my mother wearing a caftan as the center pendant. A photo of my father smiling, also wearing a caftan, was hot-glued to the upper right corner, like the cornerstone he was. Every member of my family was somewhere in this work of art.

This weaving is something I would save if my house were burning. I would carefully gather it in my hands and hang it again if an earthquake shook it down. I would protect it with my life. When I look at it, I hear my children's laughter and see the joy in my family's faces as they created this treasure. I stared at it when I feared all was lost.

I ran my fingertips along the nubby fabric, then took the stairs two at a time up to my bedroom. I opened the suitcase and surfed between it and my closet, packing my clothes for Tovya's house. I was determined to make it to our family's annual Thanksgiving party, the first I would attend in three years. I would be driving three hours away from the sick world into the well world. I would leave Dana behind in the sick world, in the care of my neighbor Elana. The people in the well world were my family, but they lived in a strikingly different reality than I did. I had been living in the sick world for so long that I felt like a foreigner in the well world. I spoke a different language.

My chest ached. Holidays had all melted away, along with social engagements, dinners with friends, and any other remnant of our life before Lyme. The previous year, wearing new dresses, Dana and I had gotten in the car to drive to our family Thanksgiving, and I thought for a moment that we were actually going to join the well world. We made it as far as the first exit on the freeway before Dana began moaning in pain, so we turned around and went home. Her symptoms destroyed any possibility of being with family.

The next morning, as I rolled onto the 101 freeway pushing seventy-five, my throat opened and I expelled a loud raspy sound, howling until I emptied out. The road stretched on in front of me, and as I drove north, I glanced periodically over my left shoulder to catch glimpses of the still, blue-green ocean. I was soothed by the bland acoustic guitar music playing on my CD, over and over again. I wasn't sure how I would act when I got there, but I was excited to see my sisters.

In some ways Jain was more like me than anyone else on the planet. We came from the same childhood, and though every child's experience is different, even in the same family, there were universal truths we both understood. Spirituality was a part of our lives, radical honesty was at the depth of our relationship, and the love between us was unconditional. The youngest of us three, fair-haired like me, but taller and chestier, she was bold, capable in business, and fragile in love. Jain could sense my need even before I knew I needed someone to lean on. She had been my rock from the beginning of Dana's illness. She called me every day on her way home from work. Knowing she would be there helped me make it to the end of the day.

Tovya was the oldest and tallest of us three, with long, thick brown hair, real woman's hips, and a flair for social conversation. When I had to sell my home to downsize, she spent a very long day helping me host a garage sale. Tovya could talk anyone into a headboard, a light fixture, or a used jacket. She took over hosting Passover dinner for the family when I couldn't do it anymore. As mothers, we shared a deep unspoken bond.

I arrived in the salty air of Cayucos and checked into my room at the Beach Inn. It was a palace away from the sick house. The white bed had a fluffy goose-down comforter. I was instantly seduced by the well world. I felt rescued. I was on a vacation from daily hell. My heart wanted to leap but stayed contained in the small prison of my chest. I unpacked my romance novel and a special quartz crystal and placed them on the oak nightstand. I put my shirts and pants in the drawers, hung my blue satin dress for Thanksgiving, and unrolled a yoga mat on the floor at the foot of the bed.

Then I drove the five minutes to Tovya's vacation house. Walking in, I smelled curry; we were having Thai food, a prelude to our traditional turkey dinner the next day. Arms wrapped around me as I was serially hugged by Jain, Steven, Sarelyn, Robert, Harry, Rachelle, and Tovya, who were all deep in the kitchen clustered around the steaming stove. There were more people together in that one room than I had seen in years.

We all gathered around my computer at the dining table, connecting via Skype to Cayla, who was in Senegal. She appeared on the screen and together we shouted, "Hello! Happy Thanksgiving!"

"Hi, everyone! Happy Thanksgiving!"

Tovya and I looked at each other, eyebrows raised. *Oh my goodness, where's her hair?*

"I'm *so* excited to see everybody. I'm homesick for a real Thanksgiving. I got to eat turkey and pumpkin pie here with the American girls."

"Hey Cayla, you've cut your hair . . . short!"

"Yes, I just got a buzz cut from the local barber! See the star over here on the side of my head?" She proudly pointed and modeled the starburst etched into the quarter inch of hair she had left.

My eyebrows were still raised. *That's my Cayla, so boldly artistic.* "Wow! You look great. I love the big earrings!"

⋯⋯⋯⋯⋯⋯⋯⋯⋯

I was back at the hotel asleep, encased in the fluffy comforter, when Dana's hysterical phone call woke me at 2:00 a.m. The pitchy tone in her voice instantly put me on high alert.

"Mom! I have sharp pains in my head! I'm so sensitive to everything! It's unbearable and I'm having trouble breathing. My head feels like it's bulging on the right side."

I took a breath to collect myself, while focusing on the smooth crown molding that defined the perimeter of the room.

"Honey, we have to call your doctor. I'll call her. Hang in there, sweetie."

"Okay, and Mom, it hurts where my liver is supposed to be."

I turned on the lamp next to the bed and punched in the doctor's personal cell number. I began to sweat. "Dr. Loan, this is Anna. So sorry to call you at this hour, but I'm out of town, away from Dana tonight, and she's having terrible pain!"

"What's the problem?"

"Her head hurts and it's hard for her to breathe. She also said her belly hurts where her liver is."

"I'll need to talk to Dana. Can someone take her to the emergency room?"

Emergency room! I was paralyzed by these two words.

During crises with Dana it was always up to me, alone, to decide whether this was the moment I took her to the emergency room. It terrified me. There wasn't any way for me to know if she would be worse off in the emergency room with doctors who knew little about Lyme disease and could unknowingly give her something that would aggravate her symptoms and make her feel worse.

Dr. Loan said, "I'm wondering if I should order an ambulance to take her to the emergency room. I'll call you back after I speak with her."

I was three hours away from Dana and practically useless. I waited in a stupor, my mouth dry, and my chest tight. I noticed the quaint dormer window cut into the wall facing the main street of the town. It was pitch black outside. I couldn't move. The phone rang.

"Hi, Mom."

"Dana, did you talk to Dr. Loan?"

"Yes, she thinks I should go to the emergency room because I said my head is bulging. I told her it isn't really bulging on the outside, but it feels like it is on the inside. There's so much pressure on the right side and I'm scared."

"Okay, try to stay calm. I'll call her and let you know what to do."

I punched in Dr. Loan's number again. "Hi, Dr. Loan. What do you think is the best thing to do tonight?"

"Let's wait it out. At first I thought she needed to go to the emergency room when she said her head was bulging, but I think the pressure will subside now that I've decided to take her off all medicines for a week. Let's give her body a chance to settle down. After that we can start with two new IV medicines, four days a week. It'll be a new IV protocol."

"Okay. And thank you so much for being available in the middle of the night." My voice was shaky. I stifled a sob. To regain my sense of equilibrium, I counted the knobs on the dresser. There were two on each drawer.

I called Dana. "Honey, there isn't anything to do tonight. Go back to sleep and rest tomorrow. You're not supposed to take any medicine for a week." I stayed on the phone with her another forty minutes until she felt okay by herself, then, like a boulder landing in sand, I collapsed on the bed and fell asleep immediately.

In the morning I got into the oval tub I'd filled with hot water and rose oil. My cell phone rang, putting me instantly on high alert.

I answered, "Dana, are you okay?"

It was Gertie, an old friend I hadn't spoken with for years. We had been close friends when our kids were in elementary school together. I heard myself carry on a conversation, listening as she caught me up on her husband, sister, and kids. I told her Dana had been ill. There was a long pause.

She said, "I'm sorry."

I watched the ripples in the bath water as steam rose into the air. We wished each other a happy Thanksgiving.

I stepped out of the bath and whipped the towel around my body. I was raging inside. My poor daughter. The IV antibiotics were so dangerous. I stomped around the room in my bare feet until the room started spinning. Eventually the gray geometric patterns stopped going by under me. I sat on the floor. *What if it ends today?*

I managed to arrive at Tovya's in time for breakfast with the family. By this time they all knew what had happened during the night. Sitting on a wooden chair at the breakfast table, I felt like I was looking through gauze. I watched pancakes go into mouths and listened to the pleasant chatter without really hearing it. I tried to smile. Everything felt vaguely unfamiliar. I hadn't seen a pancake in years. I was a fish out of water in the family milieu, but I needed this day before I returned home.

"Anna, how is Dana now?"

"She's resting and will call me later. I'll decide then if I'm going back today."

I became aware of the pit of my stomach, the dry, empty feeling there, the hard, desertlike clay. I gazed into the hand-picked wildflower weeds in the glass vase at the center of the table. My stepfather and mother were showing photos from their recent trip to the "Stans": Tajikistan, Turkmenistan, Uzbekistan, and Kyrgyzstan.

"This is when your mother and I ate a delicious meal of rice and lamb with pomegranate seeds and wonderful spices." His voice drifted in and out. I had no idea where most of these places were and had no interest in going to any of them.

I heard Tovya comment, "Robert, you're taking so long to go through the pictures."

He replied, "Yes, I have it programmed on slideshow, but I don't know how to control the timing."

His phone rang. He put it on speaker and answered loudly, "Hello!"

Jain admonished, "Robert, turn down your phone or go into another room. It's taking over the breakfast conversation."

Cut fruit was served on a large platter. I smelled the persimmons and strawberries and my mouth watered. I served myself a heaping spoonful.

Tovya was talking. "Yes, this summer Harry and Rachelle and I are going to take a trip in a 'narrow boat' on the English canals. The canals were used in the eighteenth century to transport goods and raw materials. Now you can rent a boat with its own kitchen and tour England's quaint towns."

I had nothing to contribute. I peeled a fresh orange. I watched my niece Rachelle eat strawberries. It was a familiar torture, the one I felt when I observed teens who had healthy bodies, teens who were able to enjoy activities like boating, skiing, hiking, swimming, dancing, martial arts, skipping, and jumping for joy. My Dana lay on the couch, working hard just to get through the day. I craved the life we were not having. I sat inside the sick world while the well world taunted and beckoned me. *What am I doing with my life?* I shifted uncomfortably in my seat, the buttons on the chair cushion digging into my rear end.

I heard myself say, "The fruit is delicious, Tovya. Thank you for making breakfast."

I was exhausted from administering treatments, praying for cures, wishing and waiting, as years went by. *My life is nothing like my family's lives.* During the times when Dana was able to rest, I occupied myself by painting my toenails, trimming dead leaves off plants, picking up clothes off the floor, blow-drying my hair—anything to remind myself of normal. But in the stillness, I always felt the angst of living with discomfort, uncertainty, imperfection, murkiness, and heartache.

Later, when I talked to Dana, she said she was a little better and would ask Elana to stay with her during the day.

I decided I would stay for Thanksgiving dinner and drive home the next day. I told myself the storm was over; Dana was off the drugs. I stayed, trying to keep the guilt at bay. I hoped to feel thankful at Thanksgiving dinner. I would be with my family, but my daughters were missing. Thinking about healthy, adventurous Cayla in Senegal made me smile. Thoughts about Dana suffering at home made me weep. In the struggle between the worlds, the sick world was winning.

CHAPTER TWENTY

Labyrinth

❧❧❧

*Our wounds are often the openings into the best
and most beautiful part of us.*

— David Richo

The sun shone into the living room where Dana and I were relaxing.

"It's so liberating without the three and a half hours of IVs and mountain of pills. We're having a new life, like when washing machines liberated women from hours of work. Thank God you're off the meds for a week."

"Yeah. I still don't feel very good, but I don't have the bulging head pain. I *really* don't want to go back on the IVs, Momma."

"It seems like your symptoms are a little better."

"Yes, I feel more now. I noticed the other day that I can watch a movie and enjoy it. I think I'm coming back. I'm remembering things I used to love."

"Great!"

"I haven't been the same, you know, since the IV anti-biotics. Do you realize I've been taking them for five whole months?" Tears dripped down Dana's cheeks.

"I know."

But I could never let myself think about it. *Brain. Damage. Permanent.*

"I'm so glad you're having these new experiences, honey. It shows your brain is recovering."

"I couldn't tell my likes and dislikes before."

"It's so good you *can* now."

"I wasn't able these last few years to explain this to anyone. I just knew I wasn't myself. Momma, I was talking to Laura and she's just been to a clinic that uses Biological Medicine. She was only there for two weeks, and she's much better. The doctor's name is Dr. Arnon, and he's written a book on Lyme treatment. It's all natural. Will you look into it?"

"We'll see."

I was ragged; I didn't trust the MDs, the naturopaths, etc., etc. I wanted to belt out NOOOOO!

But what are we going to do now? I never wanted to discourage Dana's fragile hope.

• • • • • • • • • • • •

To avoid the strong daytime sunlight, which bothered Dana's sensitive eyes, we would only venture outside together for our short walk at dusk. Her environmental sensitivities were worse after the IV trial. Even the dust emitted from a torn paper towel would send her into an allergic reaction of pain and swelling. It was a feat to leave the premises.

In spite of her environmental sensitivities, Dana was getting stronger, so one evening we decided to take a trip to the labyrinth.

"Dana, are you ready?"

"I'm coming!" On our way out, she cooed to our black kitty, Betty, "Aren't you just the cutest." She gave her a hug.

Thank God she isn't allergic to her beloved Betty. Even in her darkest moments, a high-pitched, honey-toned voice sang out of Dana when she talked to Betty.

We drove up the winding mountain road of Tuna Canyon, past stone walls, oaks, and pines, to the summit where the view opens up to the Malibu hills sloping down to the Pacific Ocean. We parked at the empty phone booth where the trailhead began, not another car in sight. Trudging up the dusty path, we stepped on buried granite boulders whose surfaces made up the hard parts of the trail. I looked out at the landscape, blurred by the fading light. Dana, with her jacket hood pulled up over her head, walked next to me.

"We hide during the day and come out at night! We are Moon Goddesses."

"Oh, I like that." I giggled.

"Yeah, we light the darkness at night."

By this time everyone who had come to walk their dogs and watch the sunset was gone. It was just the two of us in this magical wonderland. Walking by the light of the full moon, we climbed uphill, then headed down toward the cliffs, then upward one last time, finally leveling out onto an area the size of a baseball field. At the top, surrounded by clouds with the moonlight catching the odd-sized stones lining the circular pathways, was the labyrinth. It was laid out years ago, one stone at a time, by a local couple who placed them in the mazelike spiral.

We quieted down the closer we got to the labyrinth, while we both looked for an object or a small stone to take into its center. Mine was a brown oval stone. Its smooth shape felt comfortable in my hand. At the entrance there was a small pile of stones on either side. I entered first. Dana waited. Walking each meditative step of the winding labyrinth, which measured thirty paces across, would take us roughly twenty minutes to get all the way to the center and back out of it.

The farther I walked in, the more I felt ripped open, my gut filleted by the illness. My legs were light and shaky; wind blew hair into my face. *My daughter suffers every day.* I heard screaming inside my head. *Fucking monster illness! How long is this going to go on? I need Dana well! Why can't she live like other people her age?* I yearned for the gaping wound inside of me to close up. I yearned to return to the thriving life we'd had before the illness.

I gazed down at my dusty Ugg boots. My worn Uggs were me: warm, protective, and grounded. Many years ago I'd stepped into my first pair of tan Ultimate Tall Uggs, before they were popular. I wanted their softness and comfort. Ugg boots have walked with me through the decade of my life that included a divorce, two moves, a remodel, and the years as a single mother. The outside of my current pair had turned darker, the insides were still warm, but the inner soles had become threadbare.

My steps were measured. I kept them in between the stones on either side of the path that wound me tighter and tighter into the center. I longed to see my daughter breathe freely, laugh from her belly, and dance wildly. I longed to see her go to college, be with friends, and enjoy her life. Wind whipped my pink hat off. As I bent down to pick it up off the path, I felt each sharp pain in Dana's head and each of her short breaths.

I reached the center of the labyrinth and knelt down, my knees pressed into the hard, dry earth. I spotted a pearl glinting among the ring of stones that formed the eye of the labyrinth. In addition to the pearl, visitors had placed a bluebird feather, a pinecone wrapped in a shiny glass necklace, and the word *courage* written in white stones in the center. I studied the variety of footprints impressed in the pebbled soil. Others came to this place and left things here, weaving their lives through this spiral path. Young people used this labyrinth like an external tattoo, marking moments in their lives. Adults found refuge, a moment's peace.

I wept into the center of the labyrinth. It all poured out. Images of my daughter hooked up to tubes that allowed foreign substances to flow into her body, desperate needle stabbings, doctors' grim faces. Animal sounds spewed from my lips. Retrieving the brown oval stone out of my jacket pocket, I tucked it into the side of the eye. It became part of a larger mosaic made of odd bits of symbolic nature. I pushed myself up off the floor of the spiral; blood rushed into my feet. I could see the whole circular pathway that led me out of the labyrinth. Dana was walking slowly toward me, about to reach the inner circle. I would pass by her on my way out.

There were stones slightly out of line, so I tapped them back into place with my toe. I needed a clear path. I passed my two favorite stones shaped like shark fins rising up next to each other. My steps lighter, my eyes still damp, I angled past Dana, silently walking by on a rung of the spiral. My feet fell into a slow rhythm, joined by the spirits of others who had walked here. I was not alone. I exited at the same point I entered, the silence soothing me as I passed through the two stone piles. It wasn't possible to enter this place and leave unchanged.

PART FIVE

CHAPTER TWENTY-ONE

Biological Medicine

There is no magic cure, no making it all go away forever.
There are only small steps upward; an easier day, an
unexpected laugh, a mirror that doesn't matter anymore.

— Laurie Halse Anderson

I t was 2:29 a.m., and Dana, in extreme discomfort, woke me up and wanted me to prepare her aloe vera enema, which was when I discovered the ant raid in the kitchen. Several colonies had emptied out into finely constructed lines ending in a circle around the cat food on the floor. I wiped and doused with rosemary oil, a natural insecticide. They emerged through the seams in the cupboards around the sink, instead of through the front door where I kept a thick line of Ajax on the outside. They kept coming and I panicked, ditching the slow-acting rosemary oil for Ajax. I stuffed thick, angry, moist globs of it into the cracks, forgetting about Dana's hypersensitivity to everything toxic.

Dana came into the kitchen and began moaning from head pain, and I knew it would be days before she would be able to sit in the adjacent living room again. I scrubbed all the Ajax away, sprayed the floor with rosemary oil in water and turned on the diffuser, which streamed lavender oil through the air.

The next morning, undaunted, an army of the tiniest ants marched through the crevices in the bottom floor and down through the beamed ceilings in the kitchen. Dana's bathroom had troops lined up moving both ways across the top of the toilet, down to the floor, then zigzagging their way out the door. We tried wiping with peppermint oil, vacuuming them away, and finally put out bait. After finding ants falling out of my hair onto my desk, we both set out with a role of packing tape, vigilantly taping over all the seams in the stone tile flooring the landlord had not grouted.

This temporary seal kept the ants from their usual pathways until they found new ones. It was just like this with the bacteria inside Dana's body; they found hiding places and mutated to become resistant to medicines. That was why the healing process was so complex.

"I know why the ants came," Dana said. "They're teaching us to use nontoxic methods to discourage them from being in the house. There's a treatment for me that does the same thing with Lyme. Maybe it's time to consider it."

Is this a sign?

I called Dr. Arnon's clinic for information, and after a twenty-minute conversation, I was excited about what they had to offer, and scheduled ten days of treatment starting in two weeks. A miracle on such short notice! Floating into the living room, stepping delicately over the packing tape all over the floor, I tried to conceal my excitement, but a grin walked over my face.

"What, Momma?"

"I got you into Dr. Arnon's clinic! Our appointment is in two weeks! Are you ready for a trip to the Midwest?"

She gave me a fierce look, nodded, stood up, and declared, "I'm flipping the bird to my meds!" She marched into the kitchen and returned with two trash bags. With rebellion in our veins, we each filled a bag with her pharmaceutical meds and carried them out to the alley, where we poured pills into the dumpster while Dana shouted, "I'll never take another drug!"

We said our final good-bye to mainstream Western medicine. There would be no more symptom-driven lists. Every day Dana and I inhaled hope and exhaled despair. We meditated on wellness. We adopted the ancient belief that there was a vast field in which we were all webbed, where body, mind, and spirit merged.

We were both anxious to get to Dr. Arnon's clinic, where he employed the concepts and practices of Biological Medicine. I was ecstatic that a new alternative doctor would be taking over my "Dana project." *Why hadn't we discovered this earlier?*

Biological Medicine: Based on the Work of Dr. Rau in Switzerland

The following description of Biological Medicine is taken from the Dr. Rau's Way website (drrausway.com):

Biological Medicine recognizes that health is the body's natural state, and that health can't be restored without restoring the body's natural power to heal itself. Lying at the heart of other ancient medical traditions as well, this simple idea leads to profound differences between our approach and that of conventional medicine. . . .

1. We treat the whole patient, not just the symptoms or diagnosis, and do so on an individual,
   highly personalized basis.
2. We employ the latest hematological, metabolic,
   genetic and other tests, as well as an in-depth
   interview and examination. . . .
3. We go after the underlying causes of the
   patient's condition. . . .
4. We use multiple therapies to stimulate and
   support the body's own healing power, chiefly
   through detoxification, rebuilding the digestive
   system and nutrition, and strengthening the life
   forces of the body's immune and regenerative
   functions. The first two must be accomplished
   as a foundation for the third.

Dana had read, cover to cover, the bible-size book on Lyme
disease by Dr. Arnon, and she was enthusiastic about trying
out what she'd learned. At the clinic she received lymphatic
massage and Life Vessel sessions, and had daily appointments
with Dr. Arnon, during which he evaluated her progress. Dana
was treated for Lyme disease, and I for depletion.

While we were there, we took Dr. Arnon's Applied
Kinesiology course. Applied Kinesiology is a method of diagnosis and treatment based on the belief that various muscles
are linked through the nervous system to particular organs
and glands. Dana embraced this training fully, mastering the
technique. She was a star student, studying in our hotel room
by testing herself to see which essential oils would calm her
symptoms. As weak as she felt, Dana stood up in front of
the class and volunteered to use her new skills on one of Dr.

Arnon's patients. She stood over the woman, who was lying on the cushioned massage table, and touched specific points on her body to assess her health problems. Dr. Arnon smiled and praised Dana's accuracy. The whole class clapped as Dana's face turned pink. In that moment I knew I was witnessing her natural abilities as a healer.

After our first two weeks at Dr. Arnon's clinic, we received treatments one week per month, for the next two months. At home we installed a medical-grade far-infrared sauna to sweat out toxins, and purchased a higher quality ionic foot spa, which removed heavy metals through the feet. In between visits to the clinic, we continued the daily detoxification protocol, which consisted of fifteen-minute far-infrared saunas every night, thirty-minute ionic foot spas twice a week, and forty-minute Epsom salt–bentonite clay baths every day. We also took a small regimen of new supplements prescribed by Dr. Arnon.

In spite of Dana's commitment to the clinic's protocol, she wasn't getting appreciably better after two months of treatment, so Dr. Arnon decided to run a comprehensive genetic test. This test only needs to be done once in a lifetime because the results never change. The results would indicate any genetic weaknesses that might have been inhibiting her body's ability to release toxins. It would also identify a lack of tolerance for specific pharmaceuticals.

Dana's results came back during our third stay at the clinic, and they were as shocking as they were helpful. The results indicated problems with the functioning of her lymphatic system, and an intolerance for sulfa drugs as well as several other prescriptions she had dutifully taken during the IV antibiotic phase of her treatment. *No wonder she became so much worse!* Our decision to stop prescription medications was now validated.

According to thermography scans that Dana and I both had, neither of us was getting enough blood flow to the brain. Dr. Arnon said this was an indication of CCSVI (Chronic Cerebrospinal Venous Insufficiency), a recently documented vascular condition that particularly affects MS and chronic Lyme patients. If a constriction is found, it would require vascular angioplasty to open up the jugular veins that return blood to the heart from the brain. When Dr. Arnon told me this, I went into shock. I couldn't possibly be tested any further. This was a nightmare I couldn't wake up from.

Dana's body had swollen considerably, her head hurt, her body ached, and it was painful for her to walk. It was clear to us that we needed the expensive tests to know for sure if there was scar tissue inside our veins blocking blood flow. She and I made the decision to drive from LA to the imaging center in Las Vegas recommended by Dr. Arnon. There, we would get the multiple MRIs needed to diagnose the problem. Once again, we found ourselves driving through the cratered, moonlike desert landscape toward the city of Las Vegas. We passed flashy casino billboards and headed straight for the imaging center.

I sat with Dana in the waiting room, holding her next to me on the couch. She was achy and tired, swollen and uncomfortable, but ready to get the tests over with. The nurse called her into the treatment area to get preliminary X-rays of her neck. After that she would have to endure the ninety-minute MRI scan. I squeezed her hand. She left the waiting room walking so lightly I worried she would fall. The hall door closed and she was gone.

I hurried to our hotel, checked in, and prepared the room. I exchanged the bleached hotel sheets for our own, which had been washed in natural soap, and turned on the portable air filter I brought with me. I was just finishing when I got a call from the center. Dana had experienced so much pressure in her head and such nausea that she'd been taken out of the MRI after only twenty minutes.

My feet bolted for the elevator. *Too much.* By the time I reached the car, I was worrying about the X-ray radiation, the magnetic pull from the MRI, and their ill effects on Dana's weakened condition. I couldn't feel my body in the driver's seat. I was disappearing into the crisis of the moment. *Is this the moment? The one that precedes silence, stillness, nothingness?*

When I arrived, Dana was slumped on the couch next to the nurse, who was comforting her. "Dana needed a break. We can finish tomorrow."

I sat down with Dana and put my arm around her beige-sweatered shoulders. There was a faint look of determination in her brown eyes.

"Mom, I just want to rest for a while, then get this over with today so I can go home tomorrow."

She went back in. *Is it really the blood flow issue that has been keeping Dana from getting better?* Our scans would show our head and neck fluid structures in every position, and record minute blood flow pressures in every vessel in our bodies. Our profiles would become part of a database for a university medical research project across the country. In return, the university research team would thoroughly analyze our scans.

While we waited for the results of our scans at home, we made a big decision to buy the same lymphatic drainage device used by the clinic. This device employs ozone and scalar wave technology to support the lymphatic system, and, at the time, cost $11,000! I paid for it with money my father left Dana to use after college. It was refurbished and cheaper than a new machine, but I was embarrassed to have to spend this money. I told no one.

Dr. Arnon and I thought that if Dana could use this machine to get her lymphatic system working well enough to clear toxins and infections, she might be able to recover her health. At the clinic, the only time her swelling had gone down was during the twenty-minute sessions on the machine, so we envisioned a phenomenal recovery for her if she had access to the machine day and night. Dana and I were ready to end this bottomless fall through life even if it required an $11,000 machine to get there.

The heavy box containing the lymphatic device arrived. Though Dana and I were initially thrilled, using the machine at home turned out to be problematic. In order to keep the cumbersome pieces meant to stay in contact with the lymphatic points on Dana's body in the correct position, weights made out of socks filled with salt had to be used. Since she had to be hooked up to the machine all night, this made it impossible for her to move once she was in bed. In addition, the machine stank of chemicals no matter how much peppermint oil I rubbed on it, so it had to be covered in towels to stifle the odor.

Dana used the machine during the day when she could and all night for the better part of three weeks. Nothing changed. We had to face the fact that using the machine endlessly would not restore her health, not today, not in a month, not in a year. More footprints in the fathomless sand of our journey, where wind erased our steps. We returned it for our money back, just inside of the thirty-day trial period. We were the first to ever return one.

The doctor from the Las Vegas clinic finally called one morning and explained the MRI test results. "Dana's scans show healthy jugular veins and good blood flow pressure, but yours reveals uneven blood flow and a stenosis (narrowing) in the left jugular vein. You need a vascular angioplasty."

I was slammed. I could barely speak, but managed, "I'll call you back after I've considered everything." I felt vulnerable, like a snake shedding its skin. I found Dana in the living room and shared my feelings with her. For the first time she seemed to be able to tolerate my emotional distress without becoming overwhelmed. I told her I was afraid. She asked me what I was afraid of.

"I'm afraid of dying and not being here for you."

"Momma . . ." Dana pulled me into her arms and held me tight while I wept.

I did my own research and came to the conclusion that addressing the cause of the blockage would very likely be a more effective way of eliminating it than submitting to the angioplasty. After all, what was to keep the constriction from occurring again after the procedure? Dana's Lyme friend Thor had already gone through the procedure twice because his vein closed up again after the first one. This was the newest, hottest technique for getting results in the treatment of Lyme disease, but I was not a Lyme patient. What a paradox! Not only was I not a Lyme patient, but an angioplasty procedure was being recommended by a doctor who otherwise embraced the body's ability to heal itself.

When Dr. Arnon called a week later, I put the phone on speaker so Dana could listen in. Dr. Arnon said apologetically, "There is nothing more I can do for Dana."

Although her face was contorted in an attempt to suppress her tears of distress, after I got off the phone, she proclaimed, "I guess we'll have to fire this doctor too."

I sighed and said, "Yes, Dana. We've tried just about everything."

I lay on the chiropractor's table with hot packs on my spine and acupuncture needles poking out of my neck, again weighing the pros and cons of the invasive vein procedure. I thought about how fear can create illness and compromise the body's capacity to heal. *What's really going on in my internal landscape?* I chose not to hammer myself for spending thousands for the testing, but instead to value the information for the purpose of improving my health. I actually felt fine. I banished the images of the stenosis and began regularly drinking pomegranate juice, which is known to reduce blood vessel damage and prevent hardening of the arteries.

I'd become so used to being scared about Dana, I took a stand and refused to be frightened for myself.

CHAPTER TWENTY-TWO

New Rhythms

*The only way to make sense out of change is to plunge
into it, move with it, and join the dance.*

— Alan Watts

After the disappointment with Dr. Arnon, Dana decided
to explore an entirely new way of treating her disease by
investigating dietary treatments. She had become allergic to
most foods but was encouraged by the work of Dr. Natasha
Campbell-McBride, who cured her own child of autism with
the Gut and Psychology Syndrome (GAPS) diet. Dana found
out about Dr. Campbell-McBride from another Lyme patient.
The GAPS diet was designed to heal the intestinal lining, ultimately allowing for the reintroduction of a wider variety of
foods. I didn't have it in me to make anything different for
myself, so we both adopted this diet and followed it strictly.
We sipped the broths, and ate boiled meats, fats, and stemless
greens. This was our new rhythm. It took days to make the

rich mineral broths from organic, grass-fed animals. I got my first look at a boiled knuckle bone, rich in ligaments, floating gelatinously in steaming broth.

At some point during this period, I was in the kitchen with my hands wrapped around a cooked fish head, bones hot from the boiling, separating out the minutiae of fish edibles.

Dana was watching me prepare our meal and asked, "Do we eat the eyes?"

I had no idea. I deposited an eyeball in her open hand. "Try it."

She shrieked and tossed it in the sink as if it might bite her.

After a month on the GAPS diet, Dana's gut was better, which prompted her to continue her research into various nutrient-rich diets for the treatment of chronic conditions. She came across a video of a man who had been sick and dying from an undiagnosed illness and was able to regain his health by following the Primal Diet. Dana chose this diet as her next course of self-treatment.

She set up a consultation with the Primal Diet originator and authority, Aajonus Vonderplanitz. Aajonus himself had been diagnosed with multiple terminal cancers that proved to be resistant to conventional treatments. He reversed each of them through his raw diet. In preparation for the consultation, Dana whipped through his book *We Want to Live*, which details his recovery, diet, and eating protocol. Our pots went back into the cupboard; there would be no more cooking.

According to Aajonus, from his wewant2live.com website, "Raw fats bind with free radicals to eliminate them from the body." This is a major principle in Aajonus's health and healing diet. Free radicals cause cell damage. Enzyme-rich raw foods help neutralize free radicals, and raw fat removes them from the body.

We jumped into the Primal Diet before Dana's first appointment with Aajonus. It was an ordeal. I cried through the first week, imagining I would never have people over again because this was just too far outside anyone's comfort zone.

We began the diet with ten organic coconuts. I cracked them open, saved the coconut water, and mashed the meat into coconut cream. The coconut was supposed to clear toxins from Dana's brain. This took hours and hours, and my hands hurt from pounding the hard coconuts.

The diet was an all-day regimen, with every ten minutes accounted for. To aid detoxification, we ate raw cheese throughout the day, in addition to two raw meat meals, two fruit-dairy meals, and a smoothie. I absolutely hated this raw diet. I made myself do it. Maybe, just maybe, Dana would recover because of it. From his photo Aajonus himself looked so strong and muscular at sixty-four. Maybe it just took patience.

I drove down our mountain to a market in the valley to get raw organic turmeric for reducing inflammation, and later traveled down the other side of the mountain to a market in Santa Monica for raw cow's milk. The GAPS diet bone broths had healed Dana's gut enough for her to benefit from the medicinal effects of raw milk and juiced vegetable greens. She drank these concoctions with raw egg yolks procured from pasture-raised chickens.

I eventually joined a raw-food co-op where I could buy jars of raw coconut cream, raw dairy, and grass-fed, free-range meat. I had to drive to a gas station pickup site on Saturday mornings to get goods that came fresh from local ranchers as well as Amish farms across the country. When the organic duck I'd ordered for the GAPS broth finally arrived from Indiana, it got stored in the freezer until we would be able to relish cooked duck again.

When we began the Primal Diet protocol, we were eating so much detoxifying cheese we could barely pick at a meal when it was called for. When we showed up at Aajonus's office for our first appointment with our jars of cheese, he realized we were eating the large pieces every twenty minutes and burst out laughing! Turns out we were supposed to be eating only one-half teaspoon of cheese, instead of one and a half tablespoons, every twenty minutes.

After interviewing Dana, Aajonus sat her down at a small table with a computer where he used a technique called iridology to make a diagnosis of the state of her health by examining her irises, which would reflect the condition of her tissues and organs. He photographed close-ups of her eyes, projected the images on the monitor, and proceeded to evaluate her irises. I listened to him point out and explain every tiny formation in her irises.

Aajonus was in favor of letting Dana's body find its own rhythms using his dietary protocol alone to nourish and heal. So we left what I like to call the "Machine Era" behind. She even stopped using the magnet, the only treatment that had ever given her predictable, albeit temporary, relief from swelling. Aajonus told Dana her swelling would come down in two months, so she completely and enthusiastically surrendered to his diet, nourishing herself by eating raw everything, including raw bison heart festooned with a bit of raw butter, raw liver smeared with raw bone marrow, and every morning, raw milk blended with raw eggs.

＊＊＊＊＊＊＊＊＊＊

Out of the nothingness that looks like a refrigerator comes golden brown eggs with rich orange centers of life. They are placed on the table in front of her, and she peers into each one, imagining the worlds they contain. Her arm glides across the table to the right, picking up the outermost egg, larger than the rest. She cracks it open, watching the shiny clear slime slip down into the mixing bowl with a final plop of golden yolk. She thinks of all that nourishes this being into a small baby chick, mirroring her own fluids that nourish her heart. Without thinking, she pours the liquid egg into a small clear glass and drinks it all—the new beginnings, the nourishment fostering growth in a young organism, the light, the vibrant yellow-gold, the creamy texture mixing with her saliva. Her body becomes infused with new life.

She stares at the remaining eleven eggs, awakening the dreams inside. Eleven, the combined numbers adding to two . . . and she is not alone. The chick inside alters her mind, incubating new endeavors in her life. She rises up, pulled to the drawer of cookbooks, which have been put away, and finds the one with the most delicious cover. She has eleven eggs, eleven worlds, eleven ways to shine new dreams into her future. They will all be used. What to make? She thinks of meringues, custard, cheesecake, sponge cake, a frittata with vegetables, matzo brei, lemon pudding, lace cookies, or even eleven fried eggs for breakfast. She will not only use them all, but she will eat them all and remember where everything comes from.

Her kitchen is dead. There hasn't been any cooking, heating, mixing, creating, or alchemizing nourishment. Everything eaten is in its raw form. She can't wait to allow the eleven eggs to become the endless possibilities they are capable of. She decides to make each one into something different. Tying on her favorite cotton apron at the waist, she brings its floral bouquet of colors into the kitchen and becomes the chef of abundant possibilities.

······•···•ː•ꞏ···•······

Cayla returned from her travels and moved in with us. She was in culture shock again. Nothing was familiar. I sold her bedroom furniture when I had to sell our home in Northridge. The rented Topanga chalet was much smaller, so Cayla had to move into a tiny room on the second level and sleep on an air mattress on the floor. Not at all her childhood bedroom.

When she opened the refrigerator looking for something to eat, she exclaimed, "What the hell is this! *Bison heart?* And what are these gross things?"

"It's for Dana's new diet, to help build her immune system and remove toxins from her body." I was trying to keep the peace, trying to keep Cayla's frustrations from exploding on Dana.

"What are *these?* Duck feet?"

"Yes. They make good broth."

"Ewwww! It's so scary here! This is *not* my home. There are so many rules because of Dana. I have to be quiet all the time! It's all about what *she* wants!"

I wanted to wail at God. I could barely stay centered every day just dealing with the demanding uncertainty of Dana's recovery, and now my heart ached from wanting to give Cayla a normal and familiar home life. To preserve my sanity, I escaped to Pilates, and on my way home I saw an oak bedframe on the side of Topanga Canyon Road with a homemade sign taped to it: FREE. Triumphant, I drove home at top speed, grabbed Cayla, and declared, "Cayla, I found something for you. It's perfect. Come with me right now!"

We raced back to where I saw the bedframe. Thankfully it was still there! Cayla inspected the bed, complete with drawers underneath, and nodded her approval. The two of us lifted and dragged, and huffed and puffed, but it was so heavy we could hardly budge it. A generous man with strong arms miraculously appeared from across the street, and the three of us managed to lift it into the back of my car. I didn't know how we'd get it into Cayla's second-floor bedroom, but we would figure that out later.

Dana discovered a video about a woman whose chronic swelling was significantly reduced using "green leaf therapy"—drinking fresh, juiced cannabis leaves. Dana decided she wanted to try juicing cannabis to see if it would help reduce her own swelling.

"Momma, watch this video with me. This woman gets her swelling to go down by drinking cannabis juice. And it's not psychoactive!"

"What? You mean you don't get high? What's the point?"

"Ha, ha."

Our journey had already taken us way off the beaten track, and now we would be joining the ranks of those who used medical marijuana.

"Cayla, we need your help."

Cayla propped herself up in her cozy new bed and muttered, "Go away, I'm sleeping."

"Get up! We're going out to get medical marijuana licenses."

"*Whaaat?*"

"Dana is going to juice the leaves for treatment. The more licenses we have, the more marijuana we can get. Will you *please* come with us this morning?"

With her bed hair standing straight up, she aimed a smile at me. "My mother *wants* me to buy weed?"

"Okay, okay. Get dressed, we're going to do it legally!"

Dana, Cayla, and I slipped into a medical marijuana clinic, where the posters lining the walls transported me back to my teen years in the late '60s and '70s. Dana had forgotten her driver's license, so we were perfunctorily turned away. We piled back into my car and drove home.

IDs firmly in hand, we drove back to the clinic and were allowed to check in for consultation with a doctor. We told the doctor the truth: Dana had Lyme, Cayla had anxiety, and I had trouble sleeping. An hour later we bolted for the closest dispensary, brandishing three freshly printed medical marijuana licenses.

After being thoroughly inspected, we walked through a series of locked doors buzzed open by someone we couldn't see. We landed in a windowless room where the "stuff" was handled by intimidating, heavily tattooed and pierced attendants. There were at least fifty jars with dried buds, each designated for the treatment of a different ailment—anxiety, back pain, insomnia, depression, etc.—with names like Bubba, Green Crack, Grape God, Purple Diesel, Train Wreck, Afghan Kush, Chemdog, and Accidental Tourist.

A large vending machine held cannabis baked goods, and there were flavored tinctures for the nonsmokers. An informative, wiry young girl gave us a tour of these "pharmaceuticals." We bought a brownie for Cayla, who would probably never be brave enough to eat it. In the end we left in search of a dispensary that sold seedlings so we could cultivate our own plants. Dana needed fresh leaves for juicing.

A day later we procured the legal limit of twenty-four seedlings of the strain highest in cannabinoids, the nonpsychoactive healing agent. Then we had to face the problem of how we were going to hide twenty-four plants in our rental home, which was for sale. People came through to view the chalet on a regular basis.

Dana decided to take the seedlings to a local farm where we had been buying fresh goat's milk. The owners had become good friends, so one of them agreed to act as her legal caregiver, which made it legal for him to grow her plants and give her the crop. We hoped the adult plants would yield thirty to forty leaves a day for juice. In the meantime, while we waited for our seedlings to become full-grown plants, Dana made juice with the fresh leaves from a cannabis farm we'd heard about in our search. The pungent, skunky odor of juiced pot leaves saturated our three-level house, stinging my nose. We waited for it to reduce her swelling.

Dana's seedlings were taking root, but it would be months before we could pull leaves off for juicing. We scrambled for bags of raw leaves from two other growers. This yielded two ounces of juice a day. Ideally she should have been drinking three. We engaged in this experiment for almost two months before we abandoned the project for lack of positive results. She was still as swollen as the day she sipped her first glass of potent "green leaf" juice.

* * * * * * * * * * * * * * * * * * *

Dana was lying on the couch with her twenty-one-year-old legs curled up under the throw quilt. She was fascinated with the young, pioneering nutritionists who lectured on YouTube. Her bright, inquisitive mind sought knowledge even as her weak body required daily treatment and support. She watched a video of Daniel Vitalis lecturing on the indigenous human. Her forehead was pale and her hair was tied up in a bun, the way she wore it during the ballet years. I was in the kitchen preparing vegetables for the juicer. When I closed my eyes, she was still fifteen, thin, beautiful, and dancing passionately in a black leotard and pink tights. I finished chopping the carrots and washing the greens.

"Mom, he's talking about what vegetables were like in the wild before people cultivated them. An eggplant was originally a small berry!"

Will nutrient-dense food bring health to my daughter? I flashed back to our trips down to Mexico for the ozone treatments. I wondered if what we were doing now would end up being as unsatisfying. Fear swelled and then receded like the foam edge of a wave reaching sand. We were attempting to make sense out of something that refused to follow any known path. Unlike some whose Lyme disease responded to antibiotics or herbal alternatives, Dana had to keep searching. She was now part of a select group of people with chronic Lyme who kept moving on. We knew these people. We'd sat with them at clinics and talked with them on Facebook. They were our community, warriors seeking wellness. I reached for pleasant thoughts. I wouldn't surrender to fear. I breathed in love, breathed out fear, and continued to practice carrying on with faith.

••••••••••⁙••••••••

Our organic, fresh-harvested, carefully milked, grass-fed nutrition morphed into a happy blend of cooked and raw food as we abandoned the Primal Diet. We'd been on it for well over two months without any reduction in Dana's swelling. She was done. The diet had been good for Dana, she seemed stronger, but now she was in love with the Nourishing Traditions diet based on Weston A. Price's work. Everything we'd learned was coming together into a balanced and delicious nutrition. This was a way of life I knew I could love and sustain.

We got out the pots and pans again. We sipped bone broths, soaked grains, put butter on everything, added sauerkraut, hung cheesecloth with sour goat milk, scooped raw yogurt, drank raw milk, cooked our eggs and grass-fed beef, chopped our salads, sliced our fruit, and composed meals that looked like works of art.

··········꙳··········

Along with two friends we'd met at the Biological Medicine clinic, we joined a group of thirty people for a Lyme class, which took the form of a weekly conference call. Arthur, the inventor of this cell healing modality, had told us that because Dana's case was so advanced, she would need to be in class for a year. Arthur developed this esoteric energy healing system to enhance the body's immune functioning and heal the body and mind with frequencies made up of a series of seemingly random numbers and letters. We learned that the numbers and letters were not anything our conscious minds could make sense of. Arthur told us that each letter and number represented a vibrational frequency, and when put together, they formed specific frequencies to address particular pathogens, physiological issues, and/or emotional traumas.

We were familiar with the concept of using frequencies for healing the body, having used machines that emit frequencies produced by microelectrical currents, or scalar waves, to permeate and heal the physical body. With cell healing, Arthur influenced the immune system to return to a state of optimal functioning. Arthur encouraged us and the other members of the Lyme class to share our gains, hopes, and frustrations. Dana and I listened to him chant the numbers and letters that made up the Arthur modality while lying down in the living room. We were often lulled to sleep as we listened, absorbing the healing subconsciously. We believed in Arthur's work and remained diligent.

Dana's liberation of sorts came shortly after the Fourth of July fireworks, when she broke out in a high fever accompanied by an aggressive clearing through both ends of her body. Pain seized her, and she moaned through the next three days, not able to keep even the smallest sip of water down. I was beside myself, but strangely encouraged by all the eliminating. This big reaction happened after Dana had received a cell healing treatment focused on removed blocks between the immune system and bacterial infestations.

We called Arthur to ask what was going on. He replied enthusiastically, "This is good! Don't worry, the body is doing what it needs to do." Arthur explained that the frequencies had unleashed a massive killing of bacteria and evacuation of toxins.

The third day of Dana's release, she still wasn't able to keep anything down, so I took her to the doctor for IV fluids. I drove her to Dr. Botlin's office, where we sat in a little room with another patient for over an hour while fluids dripped into Dana's arm, slowly rehydrating her body. The other patient was a woman in her eighties, wearing pajamas with a missing button, singing a stream of 1940s show tunes at the top of her voice. I racked my brain trying to remember who she was. It finally dawned on me that she was a famous actress, still a spitfire! We laughed so hard at her stories, I thought Dana's IV would pop out and sail across the room. Dana, hydrated, mildly renewed, and thoroughly entertained, returned home to continue recovering from this Herxheimer reaction—a temporary but extreme exacerbation of symptoms as a result of the die-off of bacteria and resulting release of neurotoxins.

This tornado of healing had us stunned and excited—no other treatment had had this impact on the stealthy infection. Apparently, Dana's immune system was finally strong enough to rally. Ten days later there was an exciting lull in the house.

The discomforts of the past five and a half years fell away with the last sounds of vomiting and toilets flushing. Every day Dana shed pounds and puffiness from her face, limbs, knees, and ankles. I saw definition as her facial features reappeared. This was the Dana I remembered. She had finally "turned a corner"!

CHAPTER TWENTY-THREE

Where Fertilizer Meets Soil

The place to improve the world is first in one's own heart and head and hands, and then work outward from there.

— Robert M. Pirsig

"Wow, sweetie. Here you are, ready to go. It's a miracle!"

"I know."

"I'm giving you my job, but I need to know that you'll take it seriously. You must care for yourself now, be your *own* advocate, and minimize factors in the environment that bother you. And please, rest when your body tells you to."

"I will, Momma."

The day Dana left, Cayla and I packed up the house. We folded it into two piles—one for keeping, one for throwing away. Tighter and tighter I circled up the sickness and ushered it out of my life.

It was October 2012, and Dana was feeling well enough to take on a four-month farm internship in Sebastopol,

California. She was twenty-one and leaving home for the first time. As her black Honda Civic passed me in the driveway, I saw her wide-open face and yelled, "Congratulations!" I stood there, letting the movie end with this scene: Dana's car full of her belongings, gliding down our dirt road, becoming part of the distant landscape.

The movers came the next day, hauling our belongings to the new rental home in Topanga. I was free, or at least I felt that way, even though Cayla was moving with me. I was grateful to have some time with her. We were moving a mile up the curvy road to a higher elevation in the canyon. Blue with white trim, the Cape Cod–style house had tall angled ceilings with skylights and scenic canyon views.

I arrived with the essentials, arranged them, and began a new life. While I was out a few days later, I purchased a large turquoise glass bowl with gold on the underside and uneven edges arcing outward. Somehow it was calling me back to the center of myself. I unclasped my gold dagger necklace and placed it carefully inside. I had laid down my sword. As I looked into the bowl, the shimmering turquoise glass caught my wavering reflection. *Who am I now?*

I stared into the glass bowl sitting on my dark pine dining table. Its luminosity pulled me into the cavernous depth at the center. I felt depleted, barren of any accomplishments I might have acquired over the past six years. I felt like a false adult without a husband or a career. Emotionally broken but healing, I was nonetheless grateful for my physical health and my two daughters. I was proud of myself for surviving the devastation of divorce and illness, but there was no badge, no graduation with honors, no job waiting, nothing to fill the huge hole in my life.

While Dana was gone for four months, I entered a new decade. There would be no large raucous party filled with friends bearing gifts. I had lived in a cave for too many years. My loving sisters took me away to the mountains of Santa Cruz for a hiking-and-spa weekend. We slept in the same room together, reminisced about our childhood, belly-laughed in our pajamas, and ate lots of brown butter cookies.

The night of my sixtieth birthday, November 12, 2012, I gazed upon six women's faces glowing by candlelight. We were sitting on pillows around my turquoise-and-gold bowl. I had invited these special women to celebrate me, and to fill my bowl with their symbolic gifts. We were seven women together, like the days of the week, forming a complete unit. I intended to see myself through the reflections of these women who loved me. I had become a shadow, my own mirror image clouded by my singular focus on survival. I couldn't see who I was anymore. The glass bowl I bought for its beauty became a container for the treasures of me. A poem went in, a feather, deities of romance, wishes in teacups, stones from the earth. Songs from the lips of six women harmonizing awakened me to this new stage of my life. The bowl sat in the middle of the dining table with my friends' blessings overflowing out of it for months. It reminded me of who I was. I had planted a seed where fertilizer meets soil.

I hadn't created a website to showcase my talents or offer services, and I had no following. But I'd had the heroic job of standing by my ailing daughter day and night for years. It wasn't a job that could be hired out. It wasn't a job I chose. It wasn't a job with tenure, benefits, retirement, or prestige, but it transformed me. I was beginning anew, alone but determined.

* * *

Many years before, when I was just twenty-two, I began anew after college. I moved to the rural town of Penngrove, California, just north of San Francisco, near my younger sister, Jain, who attended Sonoma State College, and rented a loft in a barn. I had gotten a job as a youth counselor at the Sonoma Mountain Outdoor Experience program for kids. It was 1975 and I had just graduated from UCLA as a dance major, which was why I loved this barn so much. Every day I danced on its wide-plank wood floors, just as the local townsfolk had done in the '40s.

I found the old rectangular barn sign tucked under some weeds by the chicken coop. I dug it out and leaned it on the front of the big barn where it belonged. When the sun was shining on the sign, it illuminated the big red letters that declared: SQUARE DANCE BARN. This was my home.

My tiny loft had been built above the main dance floor and could only be accessed by climbing up a steep, narrow staircase. There was just enough space for a single bed and two shelves, and if I wasn't careful to duck on my way up, I'd bang my head on the low ceiling. Though the space was small, it was enchanting. In the morning I would wake up to the sunrise pouring in through the window I'd been allowed to cut into the wall.

Unfortunately, the main floor of the barn was occupied by a peculiar man, an unpopular psych professor at Sonoma State University. He was disheveled, depressed, and a good thirty years older than I was. He'd glance at me sideways, leering at me when he thought I wasn't looking, but I knew he was harmless. Nonetheless, I only danced freely in my black leotard and flared jazz pants when he wasn't home.

One of my other neighbors on the property, Skip, was tall, muscular, and handsome, the kind of guy who told wild stories about himself. He'd had a brutal childhood that left him orphaned. He was cocky and kind, and I was attracted to him, but he always acted like a big brother toward me. He happened to be a master carpenter and had transformed a cow shed on the property into an adorable two-level cottage. When I wanted to create the window in my loft space, he showed me how to use his circular saw.

I was starting to get tired of dodging the psych professor, so I decided I wanted my own place and began imagining how I could turn the abandoned chicken coop next to Skip's place into a cabin. I'd grown up with a father who fixed everything in the house himself, for better or worse, and sometimes I helped. I inherited his work ethic and believed in his mantra: "You can do it yourself."

Russ, the owner of the property, was always glad to have someone fix up the place, so I decided to ask his permission to convert the chicken coop into a living space for myself. A young couple who lived in the Victorian farmhouse on the property had already told me that if I moved into the chicken coop, I could share their bathroom.

On a blisteringly hot day, I walked to Russ's house through the orchard where the fruit trees were dropping prune plums. Lying in the grass, scorching in the sun, the plums smelled like baking pies. I picked up sticky handfuls and munched on them as I made my way to Russ's. The sweet molten fruit was so delicious and fortifying that I began to feel more confident with every mouthful. I stood in front of Russ's white-trimmed, red ranch house and banged the horseshoe door knocker twice. I heard his heavy footsteps clomping in cowboy boots across the wooden floor toward the front door.

"Hallo!" Russ boomed. He was standing in the open doorway in his usual crisp plaid shirt and jeans. He sported a neatly trimmed beard and kept his jeans cinched around his paunch with a wide leather belt secured by a shiny brass buckle of bull horns.

"Hi, Russ," I replied, sliding a sticky hand in my pocket, suddenly feeling shy.

"Come on in, Anna! How ya doin'?" he asked, as he led me into the kitchen.

"I'm good, thanks."

"Would you like a glass of water? Sure is hot out there."

"Thank you," I said, wondering how to start the conversation.

Setting the water glass in front of me, he asked, "So, what can I do ya for?"

"Well . . . I want to talk to you about fixing up the chicken coop."

"Oh, are ya gonna get some chickens?"

"Actually, I want to make it into a small cabin, kind of like what Skip did with the cow shed."

"I see. Sounds like a good idea—if you're planning to pay for it yourself."

I was prepared for this. I looked him straight in the eye. "Yep," I said, wondering how I'd pull this together.

"Okay then."

He chatted on about the weather, the cows, and his vegetable crop that year. I smelled cow dung in waves on the warm breeze. He gave me a basket of "real" tomatoes from his garden like a fatherly blessing and sent me on my way. I was on top of the world!

Two days later I was sweeping chicken poop out of the coop. The acrid smell made me feel like I wanted to quit, so I stopped cleaning for a moment and, in the hazy light, visualized my dream cabin. I saw it finished. Clean but simple. A rustic cabin, quiet, and all mine.

As I took a closer look, I found the studs to be strong and the roof viable, but the walls were fragile and rotting. Kicking a wall from the inside to test it caused the whole thing to separate and fall over like a thin slice from a block of cheese. I realized this was going to be more work than I'd originally thought, but I didn't care. I couldn't help stomping a fancy jig on the coop's floor, dirt flying up all around me.

I was clueless about what to do first. I asked Skip and he said, "Start with the walls. Outside first, then you can insulate and close up the inside walls. Check out the glass business in town for used crates."

At the local produce stand, I talked to the owner's matronly wife and told her I was going to build a cabin out of an old chicken coop.

She said, "My, that's ambitious!"

"Well, it just takes hard work," I replied proudly, handing her my apples, carrots, and greens.

"You may want to get some supplies over at Miller's ranch on Old Redwood Highway. He sells used building parts for next to nothing, like flooring and such." She slipped an acorn squash into my bag. I smiled all the way down to my toes.

At the OSH hardware store, I was the only woman there and embarrassed that I had no idea what I was doing. There was a sea of burly construction guys. I didn't want to draw attention to myself, but I needed help. The women's lib movement was in full swing, and we were all feeling it. I was inspired to walk the talk, to be a woman who wasn't afraid to step out of the roles we'd all been taught to play.

I boldly located a salesman and explained, "I'm working on an old chicken coop—putting new siding on it. It's about ten feet by twelve feet. How many pounds of nails do I need to buy?" I stood there blushing, with my shoulders wide. He looked at me, trying to put me together with an old chicken coop, maybe wondering why a young woman was heading this project.

Kindly he said, "Start with a pound and see how far you get."

"Okay, great idea. Thank you!" *Not too humiliating.*

Every day I moved forward on my new home. I borrowed tools from Skip: a circular saw, level, chisel, and block plane. I used my own hammer and screwdriver given to me by my paternal grandfather, Nathan, the great Mr. Fix-It himself. Nathan was resourceful, using everything over and over as if he were still living in the Depression. Once when I was staying with my grandparents, Nathan shaved down old soap bars, mixed the shavings in water, and handed me a jar of his new invention: liquid soap! After I finished college, he went through his garage and gave me what he thought would be essential for a new life on my own. That's when he handed me the screwdriver and hammer with its makeshift wooden handle.

First, I took down the rest of the rotting walls, exposing the core of the structure. Thank God it was still good. I started with the exterior siding, using recycled eight-inch mahogany panels. They came from the packing crates I got at the glass company. Beginning at the bottom, I layered the mahogany panels to look like scales on a fish. It was hard to secure a long board and hammer the nails in by myself. I had many trials with the upper boards until I finally figured out that I had to hammer in a nail at one end, then swing the board into place and pound a nail at the opposite end. As I nailed the boards, I sang along with my transistor radio: KC & the Sunshine Band's "That's the Way (I Like It)" and Cat Stevens's "Oh Very Young." I hammered my thumb, the first of several hits. Startled, I bellowed "Shit!"—a word I first learned from my mother when she was behind the wheel. I thought it was a driving term.

I saved the darker boards for the interior. I placed the straight-grained, reddish-brown boards edge to edge horizontally all around the room. Lots of cutting, lots of planing. The smell of the fresh-cut wood entered my soul. It became a memory I returned home to. I found myself meditating during the shaving, drunk on the aroma of mahogany. The mix of cherry and honey tones formed a rich pattern that made the finished walls look like a work of art.

My hands were raw, rough, and red. I scraped them handling the boards and chafed my arms until they bled. My nails chipped. I bought special worker's cream for cracked and split hands; it soaked into my ragged flesh at night. I felt alive, tough enough to stand up to the challenges. My arms and legs were always sore. I was becoming as strong and sure as my new walls.

When I looked carefully at the first wall, then glanced around the cabin to the last, I saw how my craft had become flawless. Where I began, the joints had a tiny shimmer of insulation showing through. It was imperfect like me. I didn't like it, but I allowed it. I realized this sliver of silver was the inner beauty of the cabin shining through. We were becoming inseparable, cultivating a deep affection. On the last wall, there were no visible gaps; the boards were joined seamlessly.

Sunday mornings I shopped at the swap meet in Sebastopol, looking for odds and ends. I met Bill there, a tall man with curly brown hair hanging out of his old baseball cap. He was wearing a white T-shirt and jeans. We smiled at each other while checking out a table of used tools.

"What're you looking for?"

"Just looking. Actually, I need a sink, a small one," I answered, blushing. His smile was infectious. I hoped my mouth wasn't hanging open.

"What for?"

"I'm building a small cabin."

"Well, it turns out I just saw a sink two aisles over." He pointed to another aisle and led me over to it. A calm came over me as I walked with him.

"Thank you. I'm Anna."

"I'm Bill. I live near here, just outside of Sebastopol."

"I'm from Penngrove, about twenty minutes from here."

"What's the cabin for?"

"I'm fixing up a chicken coop to live in."

"Where I come from in Wisconsin, people don't live in chicken coops!"

"I'm unusual," I declared with a big smile.

After Bill carried the trailer sink to my car, we had veggie sprout sandwiches for lunch and walked around the swap meet for another hour. After that we began spending time together, taking hikes, hanging out, and eventually sleeping together.

I installed the sink myself but had to run a hose from an outside spigot on the main house up to a hole in the wall at the back of the sink. Grandpa Nathan found an old single faucet in his garage and mailed it to me. I thought of him every time I turned on the water.

At Miller's I spied two large French-paned window panels and fell in love with them. I imagined creating a bay window facing the orchard, so I bought them and had them held for me until I could borrow a truck to pick them up. Bill had a truck and agreed to help me collect them the next day.

Bill pulled up to my unfinished cabin in his vintage, bright yellow truck. This was the first time he'd laid eyes on it. He slowly inspected the cabin with his hands, then put his arms around me and tightened them into a bear hug. We were still getting to know each other, and he was gentle with me, as if I were a rare and special creature.

To create the bay window, I had to convert the cabin's footprint from a rectangle to an L-shape and raise the roof on one side to change the pitch from the ridge to the end of the L. Bill figured out how to raise one side of the roof three and a half inches with his car jack. I held a four-by-four as he started cranking. Suddenly I had a horrible thought, so I screamed up at Bill, "How do we know the whole roof isn't going to come apart?" I flashed on the life of my cabin dying in this accident.

He stopped cranking, examined the roof, and said calmly, "Okay. Maybe we want to separate the rafters from the ceiling joists on this side."

"I think we just avoided a disaster!"

"Points for you, my fair building maiden!"

After some sawing, the roof was now separate and ready to lift. We went back to the cranking and up it went. Underneath the raised roof, we placed three permanent studs and attached them to the ceiling joists. We then constructed a new section of roof over the long part of the L. Not only was my little cabin sturdy, but now she was luxurious!

At the hardware store, during one of my many visits, I was approached in the checkout line by a young woman, the only other woman in the store.

"Hi, my name's Pamela. I'm a reporter for a local newspaper. I heard you talking about a cabin you're building."

"I'm transforming an old chicken coop into a cabin," I replied as I shifted my weight from one leg to the other. I felt strangely private about my project. I was buying another bag of nails, smaller this time, a window scraper, and a *Sunset* magazine issue on decking. Pamela looked to be about ten years older than I and was wearing a straight gray skirt and jacket with black pumps.

"Can I come see it? I'd love to write a story about how you did it."

"Ummm . . . sure!" I replied, but I was thinking I wasn't at all sure I wanted her to see it. Maybe it looked weird. Maybe it would fall apart.

We set a time for her to visit the next day, and she showed up looking more casual in pressed jeans and fringed ankle boots. I'd been cleaning since the crack of dawn. She liked it. Her camera snapped photos from all angles, and I walked around with her, narrating my building story: "I had this idea and just kept going with it. I got permission from the owner. I've learned a great deal building this, including how to proceed on a very low budget. I'm in love with this cabin."

I was subsequently featured in the local paper in an article Pamela wrote about how a young woman built a cabin on her own. I felt like a local hero! My friends noticed the article and were curious enough to come and see what I was doing. It felt great. I sent the article to my parents. Someone thought I was doing something important.

I was a woman forging ahead in a man's world, wielding construction tools. I knew about women fighting for equal pay, respect, contraceptives, and meaning in their lives. I was becoming an adult during the second wave of feminism. Women across the globe felt acknowledged when the United Nations declared 1975 as International Women's Year and chose Helen Reddy's song as their theme, "I Am Woman."

⁕∘⁕∘⁕∘⁑∘⁕∘⁕∘⁕

My cabin still had a dirt floor. I needed to construct floor joists before I could lay floorboards. I modified. I laid new two-by-six boards crosswise, one and a half feet apart, and then attached them to the walls. I cut the recycled redwood barn flooring to size, then fit the tongue-and-groove planks together, distressed side down. This took me the better part of a week. What would the support beneath my feet be like? Would it be strong, beautiful, and stable? I aimed for this. When I entered my own home, I wanted to experience the air sweet, the walls appealing, the roof protective, and the floor sturdy and supportive.

I couldn't wait to move in, to know what it felt like to inhabit something that had become part of me. When the floor was finally finished, I decided to spend the night. I climbed up on the roof and covered it with a tarp secured with rocks, in case of rain. I brought in a mat and sleeping bag for the night. There was a soft wind coming through the window holes. The owls hooted and the wind picked up as I fell asleep.

In the middle of the night, a wet patch on my face awakened me. It was raining. *Holy shit!* I had to protect the floor from buckling. I climbed up on the roof and found myself in a dance with the wind, the darkness, and the coal tar I was using to seal up the leak. I was pissed and scared I'd slip off the roof or crash through. What if it didn't support my weight while I struggled to patch the leak? All I could think about was the floor I'd just completed and how it wasn't sealed yet. It was raw and vulnerable. The tarp was flapping with the wind, and I was moving the rocks around to hold it. I made it down the ladder and back into my sleeping bag, wet but relieved that I was there for my newborn floor.

I used a small floor sander to make the floor smooth. It looked like heartwood, a deep reddish brown. It made me think of bearskin, warm and comforting. When I varnished it, a radiating luster appeared. I felt like I was standing on gold. Skip helped me haul the wood stove inside to its place near the sink, and I piped it through a circular hole in the roof. Climbing onto the roof again, I used more tar to fill cracks and seal around the stovepipe.

The tar looked like black worms crawling all over the roof. It was watertight but not pretty. Fortunately, I would probably be the only one to see it up close. I would have to check it periodically because tar can harden and crack, losing its water seal. I thought about the responsibilities I had now. I needed to care for my safety while lighting a fire in the wood stove. I trusted that I'd set up these things well, but from now on, I had to pay attention to my home and let it pay attention to me.

The cabin needed a proper front door. How should the cabin present herself? How should I? The front door was important. It was an entryway, the gateway to my life ahead. Again, Miller's came through with a solid wood door, just the right size. I sanded it down, and Bill helped me hang it on new hinges. It swung inward smoothly and closed tight. It could stay open, letting the fresh air in, or closed, keeping the heat and the smell of sautéing onions in.

I hung up my pots, pans, and spatulas, and arranged my records, which were stacked under the small record player in the living area: Richie Havens, Cat Stevens, Townes Van Zandt, Simon & Garfunkel, the Beatles, Joni Mitchell, Gordon Lightfoot, the Moody Blues, and Grateful Dead. The cabin was practically ready for my life. There would be music and lovemaking, cooking, dancing, and writing in my journal.

My used refrigerator was installed outside the back of the cabin by the vegetable garden and got its own overhang to protect it. Bill, who was an electrician by trade, wired the cabin for electricity. I watched him make holes in the wood panels and thread the wires through, like sewing vitality into the cabin to create light. Excitement welled up in me. He fiddled with the light switches and electrical sockets, while I settled in the one chair, reading *Zen and the Art of Motorcycle Maintenance*. A while later, Bill plugged the refrigerator into an all-weather extension cord and it started to hum. The electricity worked! The cabin was alive and so was I!

I'd been sewing my own dresses and shirts on a sewing machine I kept when a college roommate left it behind. I loved going to the old dime store in Petaluma where cotton fabric cost twenty-five cents a yard. I sewed curtains from a light, rose-colored cotton that matched the bedspread. It gave me privacy in the bedroom and kitchen area. Even though it was actually one big room, the bay windows to the right of the front door made it seem like there was a separate living room. I also made a slipcover in yellow gingham for an ugly, modern stuffed chair, giving it a country look complete with a light-green ruffle hanging down from the seat cushion.

My dad, Marvin, as I insisted on calling him, came to visit while on a business trip, and sat in this chair. I was so proud of what I'd made. This was the first time my dad sat in *my* home. He motioned for me to squish into the stuffed chair next to him and put his arm around me. When I was growing up, Marvin was the only male in our household. Exhausted at times by the emotionality of all the rest of us, he created his own rules for us to follow. We knew the minute we heard his booming voice that he meant business.

Our times were so different from his. We had the Beatles, transistor radios, miniskirts, and color television. He didn't always understand our noise and how long it took for us to do our hair, which made us late every time we all went somewhere in the family car, but he always gave us hugs we could take up residence in. This moment in the stuffed chair with my father felt like a warm good-bye to my childhood.

Using soil from a year-old compost pile on the property, I planted a vegetable garden on the back side of the cabin and flowers all around the path to the front door. Tomato plants from composted seeds cropped up in addition to the lettuce and squash I'd planted. The compost pile was located on the northwest corner of the property, up a hill bordering two ranches. The phone company came out to install a telephone pole on that spot in order to run a phone line to my cabin. I was somewhat embarrassed; it felt funny to have this technology encroach on my rustic living situation, but it was the only way to have a phone.

On November 12, 1975, my twenty-third birthday, I dressed in my finest homemade corduroy pinafore and ceremoniously nailed on the last exterior board. Bill and Skip were there to celebrate. I lifted my trusty hammer in my right hand, eyeing the top of the nail held by my left, and drove it home into the board. I did this until the whole length was secure. After I climbed down the ladder with a spark in my step, both boys put their arms around me. It felt grand to be a strong woman. I was twenty-three and moving into the cabin I'd built!

I slept soundly that night and woke up to newness all around me. The sun shining on the rosy, multicolored walls near my bed, the array of pots and metal shapes hanging by the stove, Nathan's screwdriver on the top of my dresser, *Ms.* magazines and the books *Our Bodies, Ourselves* and *Zen and the Art of Motorcycle Maintenance* piled on the small kitchen table, my blue sweater and bell-bottom pants slung over the chair. I had carefully constructed, piece by piece, board by board, a cabin, a home, a safe place for my adulthood to take shape.

• • • • • • • • • • ❀ • • • • • • • •

Here I was, sixty years old and I didn't know how to build my new life. I stepped into the depths of the bathtub and sat down, waiting for an impulse. I felt the grief over the lost years. Grief had so many faces and textures. Waves of constriction moved from my intestines to my lungs, strangling my heart. I wept into the water. I forced a deep breath.

From the tub there was a panoramic view of Topanga Canyon. I focused my eyes on the nearest mountain, green bushes dotting the stone hillside; a single boulder rested on top, standing out against the blue sky. Warm Epsom-salt water surrounded me. A spot of lavender essential oil clung to my thigh, and when I lifted my leg out of the water, it blended into my skin. I turned toward the mountains again. They looked so solid, so stationary, so still, and abundant with new greens from recent rain.

I slipped underwater to a place inside myself, a place more terrorizing than any place I had ever known. This was the place I had kept locked and bolted, the place where the fear of death threatened to consume me, a fear I could not entertain while I fought every day to keep my daughter alive. I'd breathed my daughter's breath when she could not; I'd beat her heart with mine until her body was strong enough to take over the task of keeping her alive.

What had happened to *me* in the process?

PART SIX

CHAPTER TWENTY-FOUR

This Is Insane

*In three words I can sum up everything
I've learned about life: it goes on.*

— Robert Frost

It was early spring 2013, and I was standing in my small square kitchen, leaning over the butcher block island, pouring yogurt into an orange bowl. Dana walked in and sat on a stool at the counter where my MasterCard bill was lying face up. She was home again, and not doing well. I'd driven up to the farm to collect her and her belongings after she confessed to me that she was suffering from head and stomach pain and was too weak to do the farm work. And, as a result of this weakness, she had not been able to continue with the cell healing class.

Dana's new plan was to spend a couple of months at home resting. After she regained her strength, she would be off to Boston to live with a friend for a month before starting a summer internship at Rosebud Farm in Amherst,

Massachusetts. In the fall she would finally begin her much-deferred freshman year at Bennington College.

Dana interrupted my morning reverie. "Mom, I need to talk about my skin cream, the one I made with tallow and lavender. You remember? The beef fat is good for my skin and it makes it so soft and moist. I've stopped itching."

"That's great, honey."

"Yes, but now my clothes smell gamey. My sheets too. I need you to wash them."

I was still doing her laundry because the machines were in the garage and Dana couldn't tolerate the smell of the lingering car exhaust. She was also too weak to stand for very long. I looked down at the pile of clothes she'd just dumped on the kitchen floor and saw the same jeans and blue shirt I'd washed only yesterday. My forehead got steamy. Hot.

"I just washed those."

"Yes, but they still smell. I want to get that gamey smell out. It gives me a headache."

I looked at the MasterCard bill. I thought about the utilities and how much all the extra washing cost. I thought about the ongoing cost of her medicine.

"This is insane! This life we're living!"

"Mom, I just wanted to find a skin cream that would help me."

"This isn't about you! This is about me! I know you have a nasty illness that isn't your fault, but this is an insane way to live! I can't keep up with the daily crises."

"I'm sorry, Mom, I was just—"

"This isn't about you! It's so frustrating to spend all day, every day, trying to make it better for you. And I can't!"

• • • • • • • • • • • •

Beck, an energy healer who treated intractable illnesses, began working with Dana. He came highly recommended by a friend who worked with him during and after her cancer treatments. Beck recognized Dana's physical exhaustion from the behavior of her cells, which he could "see" and "feel." His microscopic observation of the cells could occur remotely and enable him to direct energy to heal physical conditions. Beck encouraged Dana to be patient with the process and explained that her body would heal itself at a pace that allowed all systems to function optimally.

He energetically partnered with Dana's body and said that "sometimes systems or functions need to be turned back on, and sometimes the body needs help to disassemble toxins and eliminate them." Dana's body worked hard to process pathogens, increase oxygen levels in her blood, diminish swelling, and reduce head pain. By April she was strong enough to move herself, her belongings, and her phone treatments with Beck to her friend's apartment in Boston before going to Amherst, Massachusetts..

•••••••••••••••••••

"What do you mean you don't have a place to live?"

"My Rosebud farm internship fell through and I'm stranded here with all my things. I'm staying at Kim's house in Amherst."

The green paint on my bedroom wall looked greener this morning. It was 6:00 a.m. and I was barely awake. "Jesus! I can't believe they would leave you hanging after you traveled all the way across the country for the job!"

How dare this farm woman dangle a great summer job, complete with room and board, baby goats, and beautiful vegetable gardens, and then take it away! I immediately started to worry about Dana's symptoms. *Will she swell up from the stress? Will she have to come back home to live? Will she have to defer Bennington for another year?* I couldn't focus on these disastrous possibilities. I compared the green on the wall in my bedroom with the green of the tree outside the French doors. It was not a natural green. A hummingbird landed briefly on the deck railing. I became momentarily fixated on the acid green of its wings.

"What are you going to do? Are there any other goat farms in the area?"

"I'm checking around here, but I'm thinking of going up to Bennington and getting settled in an apartment for the summer. That way I'll be ready for college in August. I can volunteer at the student-run farm project this summer. I called and found out about it."

The hummingbird flew off. This idea meant signing a year lease on an apartment, and I hadn't been able to plan more than a few days ahead for all these years because of Dana's illness. The college required freshmen to live on campus, and I knew that would be impossible for her due to her environmental sensitivities.

I looked up the Bennington College accommodation request forms on the internet. I drafted a letter stating that Dana had Lyme disease, was in recovery, and might require off-campus living accommodations as well as extra time on academic assignments. I emailed this to Dr. Botlin, the doctor who gave her IV fluids during the healing crisis, and asked him to sign it.

I was going to Massachusetts in a week to attend an infant development workshop for advanced practitioners. While there, I had planned to visit Dana at Rosebud Farm. She was going to be happy and serene, holding newborn baby goats, bonding with goat families, and learning about permaculture farming, her passion. She was going to be in farm clothing with dirt on her hands. No such luck. Now I had to put my foot on the accelerator and accomplish the impossible in a matter of days. I finished putting together Dana's positive Lyme results and filling out the accommodation forms for Bennington College.

I arrived in Amherst and scrambled to help her get another plan in place, as the thought of her not being able to start college plagued me. We took her car to be serviced at the Honda dealer in Northampton. I purchased all-weather tires for the first time in my life. Dana wouldn't have to worry about car maintenance for a while. The next morning we packed up our cars with her worldly belongings.

"Wow, you have a lot of stuff, honey."

"Yeah, my car is pretty much full."

We loaded her thirty-pound sleep mat, air purifier, water filter, and yoga mat into my rental car and hit the road at 1:00 p.m., heading for Bennington in the pouring rain. After driving through the mountainous Berkshires for two hours, we entered the tiny hamlet of Bennington and went directly to Maple Leaf Realty. We had appointments to see three available apartments. The first one was a gem.

"I love it, Momma!"

"Yes! It's really cute! Are you okay with the old graveyard out the front window?"

"It looks really peaceful."

I didn't tell her that the cemetery was old enough to have the graves of women who lost their lives in witch-hunts.

"Mom, look at this fantastic kitchen!"

The one-bedroom apartment was on the upper level of a small house. It was well kept, painted, clean, and adorable, perfect for Dana's first experience being on her own. I stood quietly in the hallway of the small apartment and visualized her having her own life there. I felt a loosening, the beginning of letting go.

We stayed another night at the Knotty Pine Motel. The following day at noon, the dean's office called to let us know they had approved her request for off-campus housing. Grinning like maniacs, Dana and I high-fived, then danced around the room. *What a triumph!* We packed up our cars and scurried to Walmart for basic supplies: plates, silverware, towels, and a shower curtain. We swung by the Goodwill to pick up a chair for the built-in desk. Dana waited outside since it was too dusty for her inside the store. I held up an oak chair with a caned seat in front of a window for her to see. For eight dollars it was an award-winning steal! She gave me a thumbs-up with a grin.

A few hours later we had signed a year lease. I could hardly believe she was in her first apartment. By 9:00 p.m. I was kissing and hugging Dana. I left her in the new apartment, unpacked and semiorganized. A trail of happy tears landed on the front of my shirt as I drove the two hours back to Amherst.

CHAPTER TWENTY-FIVE

Unrequited Love Soup

*My great hope is to laugh as much as I cry; to get
my work done and try to love somebody and have
the courage to accept the love in return.*

— Maya Angelou

Touch is essential to me. I had spent years in the somatic arts world as a dance and movement therapist, developmental therapist, and body worker. I'd counseled, guided, and healed babies, children, and adults with my touch, yet during the years of Dana's illness, I could barely get near her.

Except for an occasional massage, no one had touched *me*, patted me on the back, or held me at night. I was embarrassed to feel such starvation. My family and friends knew I was alone. They accepted my "relationship status" because I had been taking care of my sick daughter, but they worried about me living without love, support, and security. My body was a desert, dry and inaccessible. I was a woman on hold, my natural instincts cut off, blindsided by illness, consumed by exhaustion, focused exclusively on survival.

⁕⁕⁕⁕⁕⁕⁕⁕⁕⁕⁕⁕⁕⁕⁕⁕⁕

Aaron, a cranial-sacral massage therapist and dear friend, had known me since my children were little. He was a lean, hand-some man with a kind face and a gentle presence. After Dana went east, I started booking sessions with him every other week. I allowed him to get close to the vast trauma I carried. As professionals, he and I spoke the language of touch. I trusted him completely.

I sat on the brown velvet couch in Aaron's office, the sun going down outside.

"How are you?" he asked gently.

I am coming apart. Pain enveloped me. Aaron cautiously reached his arms around me. I'd gone years without being held. I began sobbing loudly, my shoulders rocking against his chest. I was startled by my own deprivation. My family and friends had breathed a sigh of relief when Dana was finally well enough to go off to college. As far as they were concerned, the trial was over. For me it was ongoing. Aaron knew. The shocked, frozen parts of myself that had been my protection against feeling the full brunt of my fear were beginning to thaw. I listened to myself telling Aaron about how it had been, and couldn't believe it was *my* life I was talking about.

"There were times I didn't eat when I was hungry or go to the bathroom when I had to. It was too precarious to leave Dana in the room alone." I hadn't admitted this to anyone.

"Anna, pause and take in a deep breath."

I inhaled slowly. "Thank you."

⁕⁕⁕⁕⁕⁕⁕⁕⁕⁕⁕⁕⁕⁕⁕⁕⁕

For six years I'd longed for a partner . . .

Where is my six-quart stockpot? I filled the deep, shiny stainless-steel pot with water. Alone in my kitchen I hovered over the wooden chopping block, cutting vegetables for the soup. I cut off and discarded the carrot greens and sliced the carrots into perfect rounds. I removed a sweet, brown onion from the refrigerator drawer. My eyes dripped with tears as I diced the onion. Next I sautéed the vegetables in a pan on the stove, softening them to bring out their flavor. *A man has never been in this kitchen with me.* The soup simmered, my heart softened.

I wanted a life partner, someone who knew union, who slept with his heart open, who owned hiking boots, and who smiled during meditation. *He understands me, loves what I am made of, and what I have created in my life. I wait. I want to respond, to come out of hiding, to shape the experience of together. He pulls me out of my mothering. I am a woman who makes love again. He will always protect my best self. His face is warm with deep presence. I find him irresistible.* I felt a longing in my belly and my skin, a deep desire to be touched.

· · · · · · · ✦ · · · · · ·

I was meeting my dear friend Paula for dinner at the local bistro to hear our friend Kaitlyn sing with her jazz band. Paula had also invited a man named Howard, a relatively new friend of hers she thought I might be interested in. It all sounded like a good idea, low key, an exercise in boosting my social life; however, I couldn't control the inevitable nerves. *Dating.* I thought I could conquer the inner excitement and anxiety with the right outfit, and planned to devote an hour to figuring out how I wanted to be dressed when I walked into the restaurant.

I soaked in the bath and felt calm and relaxed but dreaded getting out to prepare for the evening. I had embraced the life of a writer-yogi-hiker, and some days colorful flannel jammies were all I needed. While luxuriating in the tub, the phone rang.

"My boyfriend says that the most important thing is to come as yourself." Paula's shiny voice cheered me on.

"Okay then. I guess I'm ready—I'll just get out of the tub and come as I am."

Her laughter cut through my thick angst.

I stared at the neatly hanging blouses, skirts, dresses, and jackets. They began to blur. I couldn't remember what went with what, what still fit, what I liked, or what felt good. I didn't really know who I was or who I wanted to be that night. Should I dress in Topanga Goddess wear: Frye boots, long skirt, and flowy top? Or sophisticated casual: sleek dress, ankle boots, and chunky jewelry? Or go sexy with a shorter skirt, slim shapely legs showing, hair up, cute jacket, scarf, and long earrings? I *was* sexy, but not overdone. I was worldly and cosmopolitan, yet earthy and natural. *What version of myself do I want to showcase?*

I decided to try things on slowly and walk out with the one that felt the best. Pieces of clothing went on and came off, landing in a pile on the bed. Then I put on a black pencil skirt with a small slit in the back hem, added a thin, green silk, shimmery blouse, black leggings, and hip black ankle boots with three-inch heels. I was dressed down, and up. I'd done it. I left with two coat options and a scarf. It was cold out. I was driving down the long winding road toward the town of Topanga, when I remembered that during the creation of my outfit I hadn't chosen an essential inner layer.

Good news, no panty line! I had a secret. A spicy, daring one that initiated me into my new, joyous, risk-taking life. I was dressed for a hot encounter with a man I couldn't resist, leaving little in the way of our having wild and crazy sex. What else could I dare to want after seven years? The corner of my mouth pulled up slowly and a raw cackle filled the car. I was going out, that was for sure.

I entered the restaurant and spied Paula and Howard sitting next to each other in the back, chatting and laughing. I waltzed in, my secret inspiring a sway in my hips, greeted them both, and sat down across the table. I was introduced to Howard, then they picked up where they'd left off, without including me. I focused on the restaurant, the comfy chairs, the paintings on the walls with titles and prices. The ambiance was cozy and the lighting low. It was obvious to me that I was there to check Howard out, but was he there to check me out? He really seemed to like Paula. I began to feel numb. If I wasn't careful, I would shut down entirely. Was there no chemistry at all between Howard and me? I was so out of practice.

The three of us discussed the menu and I said, "I'm having the salmon."

"You should ask if it's farm raised. I read that most restaurant fish is. Wild is the only fish worth eating." Howard stared at me.

Now I felt like I couldn't order the fish I wanted unless I threw caution to the wind and showed myself to be out of touch with concerns over toxic fish. His face was paper thin. *Is mine?*

He practiced yoga and told us: "I believe one needs to practice every day."

Is he telling us what to do? Is it nerves? Is he really this controlling?

Paula related a story about how she tried a hot yoga class and felt it was more of a physical workout than a body-mind-spirit experience. I smiled and added that I did yoga too. Howard looked distracted. *I've practiced Kundalini Yoga for twenty-six years. I've taken two teacher trainings. I've taught yoga!*

Searching for some way to open up a conversation with Howard, I switched the topic again, "So Howard, where in Topanga do you live?"

"I'm over by the State Park."

"Oh, that's lovely! And so convenient for taking walks. I live up by Tuna Canyon Road. I have a gorgeous view of the canyon from my deck."

"Your view is flat. Mine faces west and is very mountainous. So pretty."

My view is not flat! Oh my God, I can't believe I'm in a pissing match with this jerk. I better not speak. I wanted to leap across the table and get him in a choke hold.

"The sunsets have been beautiful lately," Paula chimed in.

Smiling through gritted teeth, I asked, "Howard, do you have any pets?"

"Yes, I have a cat."

"I have a cat too. I keep her indoors because of the coyotes."

"Too bad. Cats hate to be caged up indoors. My cat is self-sufficient—he stays outside."

I bit my tongue. *Argh! Has he asked me anything about myself? Have I missed something?*

Kaitlyn was cooing cool jazz tunes with a great backup band playing keyboards and acoustic bass. I was thankful that the delicious *farm-raised* salmon and good music were rescuing me from wrestling with this man *not* of my dreams.

"I wish she would really cut loose. All her songs are the same."

I imagined I was tied to the chair, for my own good. I clenched my fists under the table. We were the antimatch. I had no compassion for this uptight, controlling, judgmental little man.

"It sure is nice to be out with two beautiful ladies."

What! Too little too late.

The waiter came to our table and asked, "Would you like to order dessert?"

Howard replied, "No, thank you. I don't eat sugar."

Oh, that's a big surprise!

Paula said, "Oh, none for me, thanks. I ate a bag of chocolate chip cookies an hour before dinner." She smiled and explained, "I was *so* hungry."

I slapped the menu down, beamed up at the waiter, and said loudly, "I'll have the Molten Chocolate Lava Cake, no extra spoons."

EPILOGUE

Diary

❖

Life gives you exactly what you need to awaken.
— T. Scott McLeod

It was January 19, 2014, and I was back in bed after doing my early morning meditation. I checked my phone for messages . . . nothing. Then out of boredom, or so I thought, I was drawn to the Facebook app Cayla installed. I *never* go on Facebook. I touched it with my finger and it opened to a message for me from someone I didn't know named Maggie. She was looking for a Leslie Ann Wager. *What?* This was the name I was born with but hadn't used since college, when I took my middle name Ann and my Hebrew name Hannah and became Anna.

> *Hi Anna,*
> *I am trying to track down someone by the name of Leslie Ann Wager, and I have reason to believe that you and she are one and the same. I apologize for the intrusion, but if you are she, I believe I have something*

that belongs to you. I grew up in LA, and some 30 years
ago, I bought a small diary at a garage sale. I have kept
it all these years and came across it last night. I realized
it's now 50 years old and was moved to find its owner.
You can click on my profile and see the diary in a picture
I posted in hopes of finding you. If it's yours, I'd love you
to have it back. I do hope to hear from you.
All the best,
Maggie Murphy-Pomeroy

The air seemed to expand around me. *How could this*
stranger have something of mine? I heard myself breathing. I
scrolled to Maggie's page and there it was, a photo of the cover
of my 1964 diary and its first page.

I recognized my eleven-year-old self's handwriting,
embellished with long stems and curlicues. I wanted to be
graceful, beautiful, and grown-up. That was how I wrote in my
little diary with the red vinyl cover embossed with a girl in a
pink dress and pink hair in a ponytail. I had a ponytail too. Her
left hand was up in the air holding a string with the key on it
just above the diary's actual lock. I remembered feeling that my
thoughts were safe. I could lock them up.

I hadn't missed this diary. For almost fifty years I hadn't
remembered it existed. *How could it have left my house and ended*
up in a garage sale? Did my mother donate my old books and think
the diary was blank? I still had all my other journals from the
age of thirteen, when I started writing poetry.

I wrote Maggie on Facebook:

Hi Maggie,
Wow! This is very intriguing. I am Leslie Ann Wager.
Thank you for keeping my diary. I'm so overwhelmed

with excitement! I have kept all my journals, how did that one slip away? So, thank you and those who did the detective work to find me!
Anna Leslie

Dear Anna,
I am absolutely ecstatic to have found you. First, let me say I have always felt a measure of guilt for having read your diary. So please accept my apologies for that, but that feeling has never left me. But more than anything, I am overjoyed at the prospect of it being returned to you. I bought your diary at a garage sale when I wasn't much younger than you would have been when it was yours. I was enchanted by the girl on the cover and by the girl who was its author. I couldn't imagine how it might have been separated from her.

I don't know if you remember it well, but it doesn't have a great deal of entries. But the things you did write about were so significant and resonated with me to the extent that I was compelled to keep it another thirty years, boxing it up and moving it no less than 20 times and three states. I really did consider it a treasure. I think partly because it didn't belong to me. I always sort of felt like I came to have it by some mysterious accident and so it needed safekeeping. And partly because I was 11, perhaps, when I found it and so Leslie Ann Wager felt like a kindred spirit from another time, like a friend I hadn't met yet.

I have kept it in a metal box and on occasion, I poke around in that box for an old photo or clipping or some such and I never fail to stop and look through the diary each time. And so, the other evening, that's what

*happened and I opened it to the same date—January
16—and realized the book had turned 50. And that
it was time . . .*
Maggie

* * * * * * * * * * * * * *

I received the diary in the mail on a Wednesday. The priori-
ty-mail box sat in the middle of the old pine dining table with its
radiating presence. I viewed it from all angles. I wasn't sure what
would be unleashed when I opened it. *What will I find out about
myself?* I decided to take it up to the labyrinth. I carried the box
under my arm, slowly cruising the rungs of the circle into the
middle. I sat down in the center to open the package. Inside was
a present, my diary wrapped up in blue tissue paper, tied with a
thin red-and-white ribbon holding a lovely card from Maggie.

I unwrapped it and cracked it open. *I am touching the same
pages that my eleven-year-old self did!* I was handling something
tangible that held time. I didn't know then that you could write
about yourself and express how you felt. I only kept track of
the big events in my young life. The first entry was January 16,
1963, faint, but I could make out the words describing my first
violin lesson, and the stars I got on the two pieces I played. It
looked like I erased it. Maybe I thought a diary was only for
really important things. November 22, 1963, John F. Kennedy
died. I reported the facts, like a newspaper article. In my own
words, I wrote: "On this day a terrible thing happened. Kennedy was killed by a nut. He was shot in the head. He fell in
his wife's armes [sic], blood fell down her stocking, and she
screamed." I could still remember this day and how lost I felt.
"Everyone in the United States was crying!"

On January 24, 1964, I made rag dolls out of socks to
give to the children at the hospital and went to my Brownie

investiture. January 25, 1964, I sang with the children's choir at Temple and spent the afternoon at the new J. Paul Getty Museum and "had lots of fun." On February 9, 1964, the Beatles came to the US for the first time and performed on *Ed Sullivan*, a show I watched with my grandparents, Betty and Syd. "I had the thrill of my life! Every time they came on stage everybody screamed as loud as they could! Even the parents shouted!" I wrote about my Bat Mitzvah on November 20, 1965, and the party at my house complete with a neighborhood band in our garage and Mom's tamale pie. "I am now 13. It was wonderful, everybody that I knew came!" Tucked in the diary on a three-by-five-inch card was the "secret yell" of my middle school, the same one my father attended as a young boy. He passed this on to me on my thirteenth birthday, deeming me old enough for swear words:

> *Slippidy slidy,*
> *Christ O'Mighty,*
> *Who the Hell are we?*
> *Slim slam*
> *God Damn*
> *We're the boys from Horace Mann!*

My first diary came back to me just as I was completing this memoir detailing the last eight years of my life. In my diary I reported facts and events that mattered to me as a young girl with little life experience. The diary was only the beginning; I journaled through the next fifty years, exploring my feelings, wishes, and philosophies. My ramblings spoke in voices from every period of my life, reminding me of who I was and where I'd been. I wrote portraits of deep cuts, passionate loves, humiliating failures, and brilliant successes. I consistently recorded, even in the face of pain, my undying zeal for life.

When illness accosted my family, we began a journey that turned each of us inside out. During the worst of the illness, I remembered gazing at Dana's swollen neck, the size of a football player's, and cutting myself in half. One part of me dashed out of the room in fright, while the other part stood there calmly thinking, *She's growing up and filling in—it's normal.* The part that dashed out of the room knew the extreme swelling could kill her and was tormented by not knowing what to do. The part that stayed in the room was devoted to normalizing the abnormal. I cleaned, organized, and folded our life into neat, digestible piles. I knew I couldn't break my own heart and save Dana's life at the same time.

The illness began in January 2007, and in 2013 Dana was finally able to live on her own. I engaged in life again. The sun shone through my wide-open windows, warming the couch, feeding the flowerpots. I entered my sixties with grace, wisdom, knowledge, and fierce desires. I climbed out of years of shock and rediscovered the pleasure of freedom. I took off the cloak of survival and stepped naked into my life.

The return of my first diary was like the return of a lost bone. I felt put back together, reunited with myself. I relished this retrieval. My wounds and my joys had become vital beacons for new capacities. My elder self opened her arms wide and lovingly welcomed the voice of the younger. I cherished my past, but now I was most interested in capturing joy again, feeling it in my body, rising in my blood. I rebuilt myself from the original seed. I felt the wise rungs of years around my soul. I was strong, beautiful, weathered, and exemplary. I laughed openly and did not care what others thought of me.

LYME RESOURCES

Under Our Skin documentary, *Emergence* documentary
(underourskin.com)

LymeDisease.org
(Advocacy, Education, and Research)

International Lyme and Associated Diseases Society
(ilads.org)

The Lyme Disease Network
(lymenet.org)

When Your Child Has Lyme Disease: A Parent's Survival Guide
by Sandra K. Berenbaum and Dorothy Kupcha Leland

ACKNOWLEDGMENTS

I wish to thank all those who listened with generous, open hearts, and those who valiantly helped me care for Dana as she and I struggled through these years of her illness. I am grateful to the many doctors and health professionals who genuinely participated in our quest to get Dana well. I would like to thank those in my life who stayed close and held us up as we weathered one disappointment after another until Dana was well enough to leave the nest.

I want to thank Dana and Cayla for the privilege of allowing me to tell our story. Life with both of you has changed me forever, and I acknowledge your bravery in being an example for others.

I am most grateful to be a part of the author community at She Writes Press and for all the support that went into publishing my book. Many thanks to Brooke Warner, my publisher, and Shannon Green, my project manager, for keeping me on track and creating the best version of my book! Thanks to Julie Metz , Brigid Pearson, Tabitha Lahr, and Leah Lococo for the gorgeous design work. Special thanks to Stephanie Barko and Nancy McNamara for guidance along the debut author road.

To my friends: Julia, bless you for your constant love and validation of instinctual wisdom. Cecily, our loving and long-distance "visits" over the telephone supported me greatly. Jenni, thank you for being my soul support when I needed to cry under the overwhelming stress. Teri, thank you for your dear and embodied love. I will always be grateful for your motherly support of Dana. Lenore, thank you for your deep friendship and for honoring my expertise in developmental movement, reminding me that I am more than a mother. Kim, thank you for your long friendship and tremendous support. Paula and Debra, thank you for being positive about it all and "anotha motha" to my girls. Sukhdev, much gratitude for our profound friendship and sharing the joy and wisdom of the Kundalini Yoga practice. Daisy, thank you for your fearless dedication in guiding Dana's healing at a critical time. Sheri and Dan, I am blessed by your lifelong friendship and the haven your farm provides. Jaz, it was you who saw my book before it was written. Phil, I am grateful for your kindness, friendship, and guidance, along with your unceasing encouragement to continue revising and improving the manuscript.

To my healers: Dr. Hari Bhajan Khalsa, your healing touch, humor, love, and acceptance of my family extends way beyond chiropractic care. Gary, thank you for hearing my words, reflecting their power, and for calming my nervous system when I wanted to leap out of my body. Aaron, thank you for your deep listening and comforting bodywork. Guru Singh, my mentor and friend, thank you for all that is shared between us in this life and beyond.

To my editors: Suzanne Potts, many heartfelt thanks for your skill and sensitivity. This writing journey with you has been an adventurous magic carpet ride. Jeff, your attention to detail and clarity brought new light to the manuscript.

Thank you to my readers who experienced earlier versions and gave feedback.

To my family: Mom, you are a true inspiration, thank you for listening to me and loving me. Dad, I know you are cheering us on, and I thank you for giving me a healthy foundation. Robert, thank you for caring about us. Tovya, all my life you have given me a profound sense of constancy, and I am so grateful. Jain, thank you for listening to me almost daily, and for keeping me safe with your love. Harry and Steven, I am grateful to you, my brothers, for always wanting the best for us. Rachelle, thank you for your courage and honesty.

In deep gratitude for this life.

TRANSFORMATION
THROUGH CREATION

Dear readers,

Let's build a community of creativity, healing, and inspiration. Here's my invitation to you:

1. Create a piece of art, a dance, a song, or a poem about your own transformational journey.
2. When you feel complete, take a photo or video of your creation.
3. Post it on social media with the hashtag **#transformation throughcreation** and @annapenenbergauthor.
4. Tag a friend in the comments and invite them to join the Transformation Through Creation community.

ABOUT THE AUTHOR

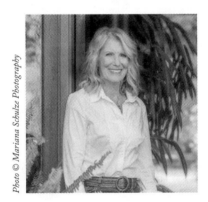

Photo © Mariana Schulze Photography

A nna Penenberg works with individuals and families affected by trauma. A healer by nature and training, her approach integrates neurobiology, psychotherapy, and wisdom traditions into personal pathways for re-patterning. Anna holds a BA in Psychology and MA in Dance Therapy from UCLA, with certifications in Marriage & Family Therapy, Body-Mind Centering®, Infant Developmental Movement, and Kundalini Yoga & Meditation. She is the mother of two adult daughters and lives in Topanga, California. *Dancing in the Narrows* is her first book.

www.annapenenberg.com

SELECTED TITLES FROM SHE WRITES PRESS

She Writes Press is an independent publishing company founded to serve women writers everywhere. Visit us at www.shewritespress.com.

Warrior Mother: A Memoir of Fierce Love, Unbearable Loss, and Rituals that Heal by Sheila K. Collins, PhD. $16.95, 978-1-938314-46-9. The story of the lengths one mother goes to when two of her three adult children are diagnosed with potentially terminal diseases.

Rethinking Possible: A Memoir of Resilience by Rebecca Faye Smith Galli. $16.95, 978-1-63152-220-8. After her brother's devastatingly young death tears her world apart, Becky Galli embarks upon a quest to recreate the sense of family she's lost—and learns about healing and the transformational power of love over loss along the way.

Loving Lindsey: Raising a Daughter with Special Needs by Linda Atwell. $16.95, 978-1631522802. A mother's memoir about the complicated relationship between herself and her strong-willed daughter, Lindsey—a high-functioning young adult with intellectual disabilities.

Off the Rails: One Family's Journey Through Teen Addiction by Susan Burrowes. $16.95, 978-1-63152-467-7. An inspiring story of family love, determination, and the last-resort intervention that helped one troubled young woman find sobriety after a terrifying and harrowing journey.

Beautiful Affliction: A Memoir by Lene Fogelberg. $16.95, 978-1-63152-985-6. The true story of a young woman's struggle to raise a family while her body slowly deteriorates as the result of an undetected fatal heart disease.